Doctor to Patient

CLASSIC TEACHINGS OF
WILLIAM A. ELLIS, D.O.
PIONEER HEALTH PHYSICIAN

Robert H. Strickland, M.S., Editor

Doctor to Patient

The Classic Teachings of William A. Ellis, D.O.
Pioneer Health Physician

Compiled and Edited by

Robert H. Strickland, M.S.

Illustrated by: Robert H. Strickland and W. Sue Strickland

Published by:

Robert H Strickland Associates LLC
P. O. Box 1388
Everett, Washington 98206-1388 USA
Phone/Fax: 425-258-6796

Library of Congress Control Number: 2016914038

Strickland, Robert H. 1944

Doctor to Patient / by Robert H. Strickland

p. 244 cm.

Includes index.

ISBN 978-0-9635919-8-2

Disclaimers

The concepts, techniques, and opinions expressed in this book are strictly those of the late William A. Ellis, D.O. **The Editor is not a licensed health professional and offers no advice whatsoever regarding the treatment of any disease condition.** This book is a historical document containing accurately transcripted material from Dr. Ellis' lectures, unaugmented personal notes, and recollections of conversations with Dr. Ellis during the period 1977-1985. Nothing in the Editor's narrative is to be construed as an endorsement by the Editor of Dr. Ellis' opinions.

The Editor's notes dispersed throughout this book serve only to introduce Dr. Ellis, orient the reader regarding his career, and point to modern resources that may relate to Dr. Ellis' opinions. **The notes are not to be taken as an endorsement of any resource referred to by the Editor.**

This book is intended for current or prospective patients of licensed health practitioners who are required by law to use their own experience and judgement while serving individuals under their care. Use of this book for self-management of health problems is strongly cautioned against.

For suspected medical problems, one should seek licensed professional care, heed sound medical advice, and participate in recommended treatment. In addition, anyone beginning a fitness or nutrition program should first consult a reputable, licensed health care provider for clearance and probable supervision.

Therefore, the estate of William A. Ellis, D.O., the Editor, the publisher, and the listed vendors, along with their associates, relatives, and heirs disclaim any responsibility and liability in connection with any actions taken or not taken based on the content of this book.

Contents

Dedications

William A. Ellis, D.O.

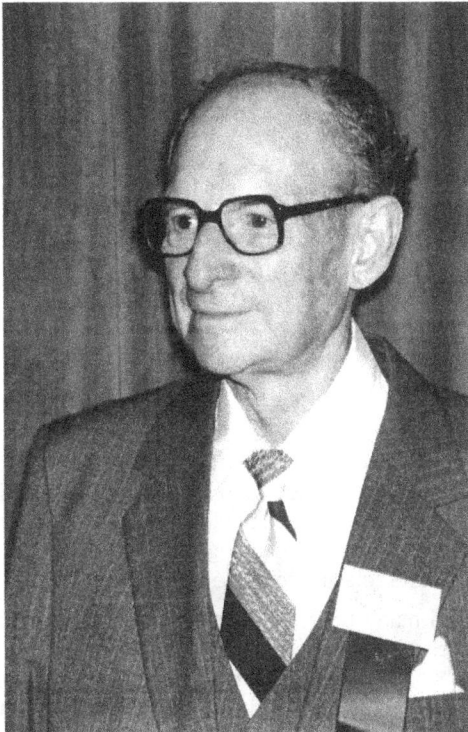

Editor: Naturally, 30 years after his passing, Dr. Ellis is not among us to provide a dedication for this book. Therefore, I provide one for him, below, from memories of our many personal conversations and first-hand knowledge of events. A few thanks are sprinkled throughout.

Dr. Ellis expressed great affection and admiration for the many people that passed through and significantly affected his life, and he was quick to praise others. Many of these are described below, and their mention constitutes a dedication. Omission from this dedication in no way minimizes anyone's contribution to Dr. Ellis' life and career.

Very influential in his life was his father, engineer/inventor Humphrey A. Ellis, a stern parent who demanded that his son display a high degree of discipline. He encouraged his son's natural curiosity and analytical mind. It was his father that inspired Dr. Ellis to start thinking about the human body as a system of levers and pulleys and the role that alignment plays in efficiency of movement.

Although he held his wife and five children in high esteem, Dr. Ellis was also a stern head of the household. Often, patients would come to his home to be treated after hours, a duty that he would accept without question, even though it was an imposition on the family. Dr. Ellis believed that he was a doctor 24 hours a day, seven days a week; and this left no time for nurturing a family. Eventually, his profession won out and he went out on his own. Although seemingly satisfied with this choice, he often mentioned that he regretted his family having to endure more than they should have. He did express that he was fortunate to have their continued love and support, which he never doubted.

Dr. Ellis enjoyed working for the Musebeck Shoe Company after his osteopathic residency, because the job made it possible for him to travel the country, treat thousands of customers, meet other professionals with which he could share information, and build knowledge and confidence for the long career to come. He particularly admired Ransom Dinges, D.O. (pronounced "din-jess") for his teaching ability and for his collaboration in identifying blood tests relating to protein metabolism.

Also, Dr. Ellis said many times that he was thankful for the personal and professional friendships he made with hundreds of other health professionals around the world. Among these were Virginia Livingston, M.D., Lendon Smith, M.D., Linda Clark; Robert Atkins, M.D., Dale Alexander, Beatrice Trum Hunter; and countless others, as well as the 300 or so practitioners worldwide that enlisted Dr. Ellis to help with their patients in the last years of his career.

Additionally, Dr. Ellis enjoyed the long-term friendship of Dolly Ware, of Ware Funeral Homes, who was responsible for bringing him to the Dallas-Fort Worth area to work, and Dr. Lois Allen, a research scientist at the Texas College of Osteopathic Medicine. These ladies rendered assistance one evening, taking Dr. Ellis to the hospital following a serious medical emergency. Also, he was indebted to Josephine Karbach, R.N. and wife of Armin Karbach, D.O., of Arlington, Texas, for providing excellent care for Dr. Ellis during the rigorous radiation treatment schedule that characterized his valiant fight with lymphatic cancer.

In that regard, it must be said that Dr. Ellis' son, Brad, took up the challenge of taking care of his father, accompanying him on trips to clinics and hospitals as far away as Mexico, acquiring medication on a regular basis. During these trips, they were able to resolve misunderstandings and build the type of relationship that they had both wanted and needed. Dr. Ellis said that he had always been very proud of Brad, and that Brad's impressive role in the last part of his father's life and the tender, loving care rendered by Brad's wife, Owanna, was greatly appreciated. She loved Dr. Ellis deeply, providing daily attention and healthy meals during his last days at their home in California.

Robert H. "Bob" Strickland, M.S.

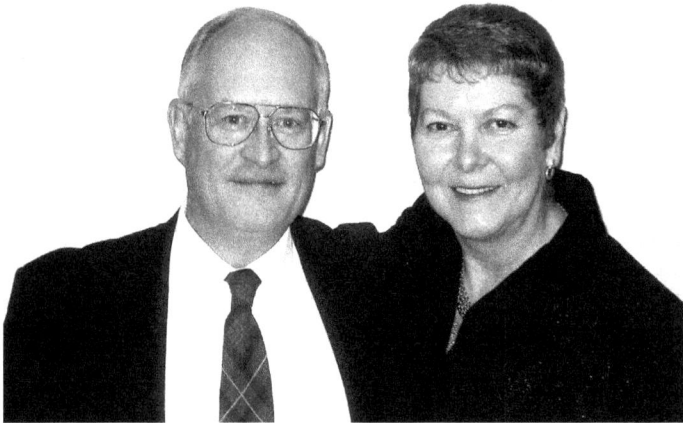

I dedicate this book to the following:

My wife, Sue, who loved Dr. Ellis as much as I did, but who let me finish his book in my own time. Dr. Ellis and I began collaborating on the book in 1984; this was right before he began a struggle with a fatal illness. When he passed away, the wind went out of my sails, so to speak, and the project languished for an unbelievable 30 years. Sue never admonished me for putting off the project, and I have always had her love and support, regardless of the delay.

Pioneers of the health and physical culture movement, such as Dr. John Harvey Kellogg (1852-1943), Bernarr Macfadden (1868-1955), Gayelord Hauser (1895-1984), and Paul Bragg (1895-1976), who, even though holding some mistaken beliefs and misguiding a few followers, weathered criticism to put health issues before the people, who have every right to evaluate them. My favorite among these pioneers is Jack LaLanne (1914-2011), who made me, a 10-year old, aware of the benefits of proper diet and exercise through his television program of the early 1950's. Over the years, Jack got it right!

The great number of health physicians and other health care professionals — M.D., D.O., D.C., D.D.S., R.N., N.D., D.V.M., nutritionists, trainers, etc. — that I have known over the years. I respect these people greatly for their choices of professions and for risking their careers to benefit the people under their care. May they be able to overcome any unjustifiable restrictions placed on them to achieve what is necessary for their patients.

Acknowledgements

Robert H. "Bob" Strickland

I acknowledge the support, sensitive proofreading, and suggestions of my wife, Sue — the former W. Sue Gentry from Albany, Missouri. She has the sharpness of eye, the broadbased knowledge of many disciplines, the consistency, and the desire necessary to do an amazing job. Any author or publisher would do well to have this level of excellence available.

I had known Dr. Ellis for about four years before I met Sue, and Dr. Ellis was the only objective person I trusted to see if she would meet my exacting requirements for a life partner. He gave her a strong endorsement after their first meeting — a two-hour private conversation. That was good enough for me, and, as of the publication date of this book, Sue and I will have been married for over 30 years. Sue has a marvelous perspective on the man and has reminisced with me about our times with him. Without each other, this project would never have been completed.

Those That Helped Me Along the Way

Thanks to the following people who helped me gain an appreciation of the disciplines described in this book.

To Brad Ellis, for his patience and for allowing me to retain a mountain of Dr. Ellis' personal correspondence and reference materials. Without my access to this collection, it would be difficult to impossible for Dr. Ellis' work to be made available to new generations of health professionals.

To Joe Oneal and the late Stan Bynum of Nutri-Dyn (now Progressive) for hiring me as an inside technical representative in 1978. It was a huge challenge to gear up to a different way of thinking about maintaining one's health. It was there I met Dr. Ellis, beginning a 10-year friendship that I might never have had the privilege of enjoying without having answered a small Nutri-Dyn ad in the Dallas Morning News.

To the late Frank DeLuca of Biotics Research Corporation, who hired me in the same capacity for his company. It was a close business relationship with Dr. Ellis that allowed me almost daily contact with him on a professional basis. This constant interaction provided me a completely new way of understanding the body and the techniques of maintaining it, and it bestowed upon me the responsibility of sharing what I have learned whenever and wherever necessary.

To my dear friend and co-worker during the Nutri-Dyn and Biotics years, Iola Murray, for attending to the dozens of administrative and clerical duties while I was developing materials for Biotics, learning from Dr. Ellis, helping the outside sales force, and fielding the many calls that occurred throughout the day. Her talent and dedication puts her among the very best.

To Lew Hulvey, D.C. of Judsonia, Arkansas, for 37 years of friendship, support, and advice from his personal standpoint; it is remarkable how congruent his beliefs about health are with those of Dr. Ellis.

To Denis DeLuca, Bill Sparks, and the rest of the folks at Biotics Research Corporation for an ongoing personal and professional friendship spanning more than 35 years. Their products are thoughtfully formulated, manufactured under highly sanitary conditions, and of consistently high quality. Their products make sense from a scientific standpoint and continue to be at the core of my and my wife's supplement regimen, which we both hope to enjoy into a very productive old age.

Those Who Provided Direction and Materials

Thanks to the following who made their own significant contributions to the book.

Alan Cantwell, M.D.
Aries Rising Press
PO Box 29532
 Los Angeles, CA 90029
(www.ariesrisingpress.com)
Email: alancantwell@sbcglobal.net.

Lynn Donches, Chief Librarian
Rodale Library
400 South Tenth Street
Emmaus, PA 18098-0099
Phone: 610-967-8729

Owanna Ellis for providing a picture of William A. Ellis, D.O. ("Bampi" to his family)
Picture courtesy of the Consumer Health Organization of Canada, taken on Friday, March 30, 1985 at the Total Health '85 Convention in Toronto, the last convention that Dr. Ellis attended.

Helen Faria, Admin
Former Managing Editor, *Medical Sentinel*
http://www.haciendapub.com/medicalsentinel
The official, peer-review journal of the Association of American Physicians and Surgeons (AAPS). The *Medical Sentinel* is committed to publishing scholarly articles in defense of the practice of private medicine, the tenets and principles set forth in the Oath of Hippocrates, individually-based medical ethics, and the sanctity of the patient-doctor relationship.

David Forgie, D.C., and Grant Bjornson, D.C. for providing a very important transcript of Dr. Ellis' lecture and demonstration for the Alpha Chi Beta group at Canadian Memorial Chiropractic College, Toronto, Ontario, Canada, December 2-4, 1977.
Dr. Forgie: http://www.rothesaychiropractic.ca
Dr.Bjornson: http://www.canpages.ca/website/business/
210701?website=http%3A%2F%2Fbobcaygeonchiropractic.ca%2F

David H. Freedman
c/o Atlantic Media Company
600 New Hampshire Ave., NW
Washington, DC 20037

Oneta Hansen for providing a picture and history of her father, Ransom Dinges, D.O.

Debra Loguda-Summers, Curator/Special Projects
Museum of Osteopathic Medicine, SM
and International Center for Osteopathic History
800 West Jefferson
Kirksville, MO 63501
Toll Free: 1 866 626 ATSU Ext. 2359

Wes Miller
Foot-So-Port Shoe Company (formerly Musebeck and Health Spot companies)
Oconomowoc Business Center
405 E. Forest Street
Oconomowoc, WI 53066

Robyn Oro, Cataloging Assistant
D'Angelo Library
Kansas City University of Medicine and Biosciences
1750 Independence, MO 64106-1453
Phone: 816-654-7267

Steve Zoltai, Collections Librarian & Archivist
CMCC Health Sciences Library
Canadian Memorial Chiropractic College
6100 Leslie Street
Toronto, ON M2H 3J1
(416) 482-2340 x206

Pixabay
Braxmeier & Steinberger GbR (VAT Reg.No.: DE297456622),
Hans Braxmeier, Donaustraße 13, 89231 Neu-Ulm, Germany
Phone: +49 (0)731 / 800 1660
info(at)pixabay.com (https://pixabay.com/)

Foreword

As the years pass, fewer people that knew William A. "Dr. Bill" Ellis, D.O. (February 25, 1906-September 16, 1986) remain among us. The patients, colleagues, and lay persons that are alive have probably not forgotten him, and most of them, I assume, have fond memories.

Editor: There is a companion book to *Doctor to Patient* for licensed health professionals titled *Doctor to Doctor*. It includes detailed chapters that inform health practitioners how to carry out Dr. Ellis' comprehensive program for patients. It also serves as a standalone resource for other licensed health advocates. Copies of both books are available from the same sources.

Dr. Ellis was born in New Jersey, the son of an inventor, Humphrey Ellis. He graduated from Philadelphia Osteopathic College in 1931 and spent the next 50-odd years making people more healthy. He was a large man — 6'2" tall, with a personality bigger than life — an extrovert in a bow tie, with a beaming smile and warm (size 16) handshake. The intelligent understood his opinionated manner; catching on right away that Dr. Ellis was dedicated to health, deeply studied, widely traveled, and intensely interested in helping others. The ignorant might have branded him as arrogant, but nothing could have been further from the truth. What he had was confidence, and rightly so. Dr. Ellis excelled at many endeavors. He was skilled in many sports, and one may have branded him a jock in college.

He played semi-professional baseball, with a batting average of 0.387. He also played basketball professionally to help pay for his osteopathic training, but he loved bowling just as much, with its opportunity to interact with hard-working, real people. He liked golf too, but he modified the typical, leisurely round into an aerobic exercise, covering an 18-hole course in roughly 2/3 of the usual time!

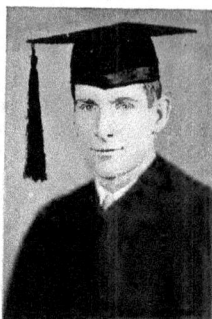

WILLIAM A. ELLIS

Phi Sigma Gamma; Basketball, 1, 2, 3, 4; Baseball, 1, 2, 3, 4; Golf, 2, 3, 4; Bowling, 2, 3, 4; Tennis, 2; Interclass Swimming, 1, 2; Athletic Editor, *Synapsis*, 3; Athletic Editor, *Axone*, 2; Business Manager, *Axone*, 3, 4; Neo Honorary Society.

Dr. Ellis had pretty rigid social and religious beliefs, shaped by a stern upbringing, but he would listen to, reflect upon, and even incorporate others' ideas, if they were plausible. He had no use for phonies, shysters, or even closed-minded people — especially when it concerned health issues or nutritional products. In his personal notes, Dr. Ellis wrote that he had studied the makeup of the National Science Board, the policy-making body for the National Science Foundation, for the period from 1957 to 1973. He found that, of the 78 scientists officially listed as "academic", 62 were on the payroll of large corporations.

Dr. Ellis was just as outspoken and critical about individuals and companies misrepresenting their products and treatments. I remember one instance when Dr. Ellis warned the president of a nutritional supplement company that he would throw him out of his hotel room. This was in response to the individual attempting to tell Dr. Ellis what to say during his upcoming lecture sponsored by the very same company! At 72 years old, Dr. Ellis was robust enough to accomplish it, and he lectured without restrictions.

What was Dr. Ellis About?

Dr. Ellis was a family practitioner and surgeon; he delivered hundreds of newborns, and he was an expert in foot and postural disorders. His favorite activity, however, was working with patients to restore good health. In pursuit of this goal, he read scholarly journals, studied anecdotal information, attended all types of medical and health-related conferences and trade shows, and tested various modalities in his own practice. To determine what disease condition was present, like any skilled physician or other health practitioner, Dr. Ellis would begin with a clinical diagnosis, assessing a patient's symptoms. This assessment, along with a review of the patient's medical history, a physical examination, and various tests, would enable him to make a medical diagnosis.

His goal was always to eliminate pathology and restore a patient's anatomy and physiology to homeostasis. He constantly refined his concept of normal, and he used various modalities to normalize patients' test results. His treatments involved osteopathic manipulations, adjustment of the diet, internal cleansing procedures, and nutrient supplementation. He considered a proper diet to be the most important consideration, with careful attention being paid to the individual's ability to digest and assimilate dietary protein. In shaping his beliefs, four individuals figure prominently in Dr. Ellis' professional life, and they are discussed below.

Weston A. Price, D.D.S.

Dr. Ellis suffered a physical breakdown himself in 1936 and began a serious study of nutrition, if for no other reason than to find solutions to his own problem. Soon thereafter, he became a proponent of the beliefs of Dr. Weston A. Price, D.D.S. (1870-1948). After 1930, Dr. Price devoted most of his study to nutrition, studying carefully the diets of various cultures around the world. In 1939, he published *Nutrition and Physical Degeneration*, in which he concluded that the Western diet, including flour, sugar, and processed vegetable fats were the major cause of of nutritional deficiencies, leading to dental disease. This book was valuable to Dr. Ellis.

Francis M. Pottenger, Jr., M.D.

Francis M. Pottenger, Jr., M.D. (1901-1967) was also a proponent of Dr. Price, and he operated the Pottenger Sanatorium, which his father had founded for treatment of tuberculosis in Monrovia, California. Dr. Pottenger provided liver, butter, cream, and eggs to convalescing patients, and he gave adrenal cortex supplements to treat exhaustion. His meat and milk studies with cats are often quoted.

Pottenger's meat study resolved that the animals fed an all-raw diet of 2/3 meat, 1/3 raw milk, and cod liver oil remained healthy, while those on a diet of 2/3 cooked meat, 1/3 milk, and cod liver oil developed health problems which were passed on to subsequent generations of progeny. Problems with parasites, skin diseases, and allergies increased from 5% to 90% in the third generation of deficient cats. Their bones became soft, as well. Later, it was shown that supplementing the deficient diets with the essential amino acid taurine could offset the detrimental effects, presumably through augmentation of protein synthesis.

Pottenger's milk study cats were fed 1/3 raw meat and 2/3 milk. What was varied was the way the milk was processed. Cats given raw milk were healthier than those given pasteurized, evaporated, sweetened condensed, or raw metabolized vitamin D milk.

Melvin Page, D.D.S.

Melvin E. Page, D.D.S. (1894-1983) was also a proponent of the teachings of Weston A. Price, D.D.S. He was the son of a physician. After one year in college, Dr. Page quit school to teach school in rural Montana. After two years, he decided to return to the University of Michigan where he obtained a Doctorate of Dental Surgery degree. In 1919, He began a successful dental practice in Muskegon, Michigan, inventing dentures based on sound engineering principles that minimized bone loss.

His research into bone loss led him to Dr. Weston Price's work with primitive people, and he started his investigations at Mercy Hospital and Hackley Hospital in Muskegon. He ran more than two thousand blood chemistries and discovered that no absorption of bone (and no cavities) occurred when the calcium to phosphorus ratio were in a proportion of 10 to 4 in the blood (2.5:1). The Department of Dental Research of the United States Air Force confirmed his findings of the calcium/phosphorus ratio to be correct 42 years later. Dr. Page also found, according to test readings, that the blood sugar level should be at 85, plus or minus 5 (Sclavo test).

In 1940, Dr. Page resettled in St. Petersburg, Florida, remaining there until his death. At the age of 84, he still walked a mile to and from his office almost daily. He believed that body chemistry, when properly balanced by proper nutrition and other factors, will not only prevent dental problems but will naturally affect the rest of the body as well. His treatment philosophy was simple and logical, as follows.

- The harmful effects of the use of white sugar and refined carbohydrates can't be ignored.

- The harmful effects of using chemical additives and other food preservatives for the sake of shelf life upsets body chemistry.
- Using whole food vitamin concentrates, minerals and digestive enzymes to supplement daily food intake might be necessary.
- Milk is not the perfect food for everyone.

Dr. Page used small doses of endocrine extracts to balance the body chemistry. When patients were in his facility, he was able to check and recheck the blood chemistry, especially the calcium/phosphorus (Ca/P) ratio, every three to four days. His Page Food Plan was developed during this time because he noticed that certain foods upset body chemistry more than others. Dr. Ellis worked and studied with Dr. Page during breaks from his practice.

Royal Lee, D.D.S.

Royal Lee, D.D.S. (1895-1967) had an interest in nutrition from youth. In his senior year of dental school, he presented The Systemic Causes of Dental Caries, written when he was 16 years old and explaining the relationship among tooth decay, vitamin deficiency, and the endocrine glands. Although a practicing dentist, he was an inventor with several patents in his name, including a speed governor for electric motors.

In 1929, Dr. Lee introduced a natural food-based supplement in the "most potent and bioavailable form", which he named Catalyn. It was derived from defatted wheat germ, carrots, nutritional yeast, bovine adrenal, liver, spleen, and kidney, dried pea (vine) juice, dried alfalfa juice, mushroom, oat flour, soy bean lecithin, and rice bran extract. The demand was great enough to necessitate creation of a new company, the Vitamin Products Company, later called Standard Process. Dr. Ellis used Standard Process products extensively in his own practice.

In time, Dr. Lee introduced other nutritional tools for practitioners to use in treating their patients, such as Phosfood Liquid in 1931, for support of calcium metabolism and sympathetic nervous system function. By 1934 the demand by physicians convinced Dr. Lee to separate the various vitamin complexes into separate products (vitamins A through G) for more precise clinical application. From 1935 through 1939 he introduced five new products: Drenamin (adrenal support), organic minerals (parasympathetic support), soy bean lecithin, lactic acid yeast (proper pH for healthy functioning of the gastrointestinal system), and wheat germ oil perles (one of the richest sources of natural vitamin E complex).

The 1940s saw a wide variety of specific nutritional products added to the Vitamin Products Company line. In the 1950s, Dr. Lee developed a type of glandular product, that he termed protomorphogen extracts, produced by a process he patented. These were not simply desiccated glandulars but "uniquely-derived nucleoprotein-mineral extracts."

In 1941, Dr. Lee organized the Lee Foundation for Nutritional Research to engage in research and coordinate and communicate nutritional breakthroughs from laboratories around the world. The Foundation was the world's largest clearinghouse for nutritional information for doctors, agriculturists, and homemakers. During its existence the Lee Foundation disseminated millions of pieces of literature and hundreds of thousands of books on health and nutrition. In 1947 he coauthored a book with William Hanson entitled *Protomorphology, Study of Cell Autoregulation,* a study of biological growth factors and a survey of the problems of aging. The Standard Process company continues to offer these products to health care professionals.

> **Editor:** See the article about Dr. Lee written by David L. Morris, B.S., D.C. at http://www.westonaprice.org/health-topics/royal-lee-dds-father-of-natural-vitamins/.

Clinical Research Groups

Dr. Ellis often used the phrases "our research" and "our opinion" in his lectures. What he meant by these references is that he was part of one or more large groups that included physicians, nurses, dentists, nutritionists, academic researchers, physicists, chemical engineers, chemists, public health officials, and allied health professionals. He was a member of the Jarvis Group, established and maintained in the 1930s and 1940s by D. C. Jarvis, M.D. Membership included many other licensed practitioners.

Members of such groups routinely shared information with each other via letter and telephone, as well as during conventions, trade shows, workshops, and seminars. Many were authors of books. The constant ebb and flow of information was scrutinized by numbers of people with critical minds who had a common purpose: to elevate the state of health of all individuals. Therefore, the information was freely exchanged; there was no secrecy. Being a member and president (1955) of the American College of Osteopathy, Dr. Ellis was aware of the value of all types of research in the furtherance of his chosen profession and looked forward to new developments with great enthusiasm.

How did a patient fare on a new treatment? Were there any unexpected results? Did the patient die? What would you suggest for treating a particular disease? Certainly, some far out ideas were expressed within these study groups, but their lack of success usually became apparent, or the ideas were not taken favorably by the group. The point is that well-educated health professionals were evaluating burgeoning notions all of the time. Was it scientific research? No; much of it did not adhere to the tenants of experimental design. Were the conclusions useful in clinical practice? Yes, especially In the absence of "reliable evidence-based results" from the study of specific nutrition-based methodologies.

Naturally, this visibility made all participants vulnerable to the Gestapo tactics of the Food and Drug Administration and state medical boards. Were some disreputable persons within these groups for their own gain? Probably; and these individuals should have been and often were stopped in their tracks by their peers. However, the harassment of honest, well-meaning practitioners continued for a very long time, with many practitioners losing their licenses. Some relief came in the form of legislation introduced in Congress by Senator William Proxmire in the 1970s.

As we shall see in the following sections, there are medical researchers and science journalists that doubt the reliability of much evidence-based research results, as published in many scholarly journals. Their reasons will be apparent from the excerpts that have been selected, and the reader may find the entire articles at the links or in the journals indicated.

The Later Years

When Dr. Ellis retired in 1972, he sold his practice in Tarentum, Pennsylvania and moved to the Dallas/Fort Worth area to begin consulting on laboratory tests to licensed health practitioners. During this period, he was a personal consultant to over 300 physicians worldwide, and he lectured extensively at various health conferences, trade shows, and smaller, regional events, in the United States, Canada, and some foreign countries. He did not apply for a license in Texas or any other state, confining his work with patients to only those of other, licensed professionals.

Evidence-based Research

In their article in the *British Medical Journal* entitled, *Evidence-based medicine: what it is and what it isn't* (BMJ 1996;312:71), doctors David L Sackett, William M C Rosenberg, J A Muir Gray, R Brian Haynes, and W Scott Richardson attempt to clarify the role of evidence-based research (external clinical evidence) in a clinician's practice. Some direct quotes from that article are given below. You may find the entire article on the Internet at http://dx.doi.org/10.1136/bmj.312.7023.71.

"It's about integrating individual clinical expertise and the best external evidence....

Evidence-based medicine is the conscientious, explicit, and judicious use of current best evidence in making decisions about the care of individual patients. **The practice of evidence-based medicine means integrating individual clinical expertise with the best available external clinical evidence from systematic research.** By individual clinical expertise we mean the proficiency and judgment that individual clinicians acquire through clinical experience and clinical practice....

Good doctors use both individual clinical expertise and the best available external evidence, and neither alone is enough. Without clinical expertise, practice risks becoming tyrannized by evidence, for even excellent external evidence may be inapplicable to or inappropriate for an individual patient. Without current best evidence, practice risks becoming rapidly out of date, to the detriment of patients....

Evidence-based medicine is not cookbook medicine. Because it requires a bottom up approach that integrates the best external evidence with individual clinical expertise and patients' choice, it cannot result in slavish, cookbook approaches to individual patient care. External clinical evidence can inform, but can never replace, individual clinical expertise, and it is this expertise that decides whether the external evidence applies to the individual patient at all and, if so, how it should be integrated into a clinical decision. Similarly, any external guideline must be integrated with individual clinical expertise in deciding whether and how it matches the patient's clinical state, predicament, and preferences, and thus whether it should be applied."

David H. Freedman has been an *Atlantic Magazine* **contributor since 1998. In his October 4, 2010 article, published in the November 2010 issue,** *Lies, Damned Lies, and Medical Science,* **he states, "Much of what medical researchers conclude in their studies is misleading, exaggerated, or flat-out wrong.** Though the results of drug studies often make newspaper headlines, you have to wonder whether they prove anything at all. Indeed, given the breadth of the potential problems raised at [a meeting I attended at the University of Ioannina, Greece medical school's teaching hospital], can any medical-research studies be trusted? So why are doctors — to a striking extent — still drawing upon misinformation in their everyday practice?" **Here are some more quotations from that article.**

"Dr. John Ioannidis, who has spent his career challenging his peers by exposing their bad science....[is] what's known as a meta-researcher, and he's become one of the world's foremost experts on the credibility of medical research. He and his team have shown, again and again, and in many different ways, that much of what biomedical researchers conclude in published studies — conclusions that doctors keep in mind when they prescribe antibiotics or blood-pressure medication, or when they advise us to consume more fiber or less meat, or when they recommend surgery for heart disease or back pain — is misleading, exaggerated, and often flat-out wrong.

He charges that as much as 90% of the published medical information that doctors rely on is flawed. His work has been widely accepted by the medical community; it has been published in the field's top journals, where it is heavily cited; and he is a big draw at conferences. Given this exposure, and the fact that his work broadly targets everyone else's work in medicine, as well as everything that physicians do and all the health advice we get, Ioannidis may be one of the most influential scientists alive. Yet for all his influence, he worries that the field of medical research is so pervasively flawed, and so riddled with conflicts of interest, that it might be chronically resistant to change — or even to publicly admitting that there's a problem....And sure enough, he goes on to suggest that an obsession with winning funding has gone a long way toward weakening the reliability of medical research.

He first stumbled on the sorts of problems plaguing the field, he explains, as a young physician-researcher in the early 1990s at Harvard....A new "evidence-based medicine" movement was just starting to gather force, and Ioannidis decided to throw himself into it, working first with prominent researchers at Tufts University and then taking positions at Johns Hopkins University and the National Institutes of Health. He was unusually well armed: he had been a math prodigy of near-celebrity status in high school in Greece, and had followed his parents, who were both physician-researchers, into medicine. Now he'd have a chance to combine math and medicine by applying rigorous statistical analysis to what seemed a surprisingly sloppy field. "I assumed that everything we physicians did was basically right, but now I was going to help verify it," he says. "All we'd have to do was systematically review the evidence, trust what it told us, and then everything would be perfect."

It didn't turn out that way. In poring over medical journals, he was struck by how many findings of all types were refuted by later findings. Of course, medical-science "never minds" are hardly secret. And they sometimes make headlines, as when in recent years large studies or growing consensuses of researchers concluded that mammograms, colonoscopies, and PSA tests are far less useful cancer-detection tools than we had been told; or when widely prescribed antidepressants such as Prozac, Zoloft, and Paxil were revealed to be no more effective than a placebo for most cases of depression; or when we learned that staying out of the sun entirely can actually increase cancer risks; or when we were told that the advice to drink lots of water during intense exercise was potentially fatal; or when, last April, we were informed that taking fish oil, exercising, and doing puzzles doesn't really help fend off Alzheimer's disease, as long claimed. Peer-reviewed studies have come to opposite conclusions on whether using cell phones can cause brain cancer, whether sleeping more than eight hours a night is healthful or dangerous, whether taking aspirin every day is more likely to save your life or cut it short, and whether routine angioplasty works better than pills to unclog heart arteries.

But beyond the headlines, Ioannidis was shocked at the range and reach of the reversals he was seeing in everyday medical research. "Randomized controlled trials," which compare how one group responds to a treatment against how an identical group fares without the treatment, had long been considered nearly unshakable evidence, but they, too, ended up being wrong some of the time. "I realized even our gold-standard research had a lot of problems," he says. Baffled, he started looking for the specific ways in which studies were going wrong. And before long he discovered that the range of errors being committed was astonishing: from what questions researchers posed, to how they set up the studies, to which patients they recruited for the studies, to which measurements they took, to how they analyzed the data, to how they presented their results, to how particular studies came to be published in medical journals.

This array suggested a bigger, underlying dysfunction, and Ioannidis thought he knew what it was. **"The studies were biased," he says. "Sometimes they were overtly biased. Sometimes it was difficult to see the bias, but it was there." Researchers headed into their studies wanting certain results — and, lo and behold, they were getting them.**

We think of the scientific process as being objective, rigorous, and even ruthless in separating out what is true from what we merely wish to be true, but in fact it's easy to manipulate results, even unintentionally or unconsciously. "At every step in the process, there is room to distort results, a way to make a stronger claim or to select what is going to be concluded," says Ioannidis. "There is an intellectual conflict of interest that pressures researchers to find whatever it is that is most likely to get them funded."

He chose to publish one paper, fittingly, in the online journal PLoS Medicine, which is committed to running any methodologically sound article without regard to how "interesting" the results may be. In the paper, Ioannidis laid out a detailed mathematical proof that, assuming modest levels of researcher bias, typically imperfect research techniques, and the well-known tendency to focus on exciting rather than highly plausible theories, researchers will come up with wrong findings most of the time. His model predicted, in different fields of medical research, rates of wrongness roughly corresponding to the observed rates at which findings were later convincingly refuted: 80% of non-randomized studies (by far the most common type) turn out to be wrong, as do 25% of supposedly gold-standard randomized trials, and as much as 10% of the platinum-standard large randomized trials. The article spelled out his belief that researchers were frequently manipulating data analyses, chasing career-advancing findings rather than good science, and even using the peer-review process — in which journals ask researchers to help decide which studies to publish — to suppress opposing views.

The other paper...zoomed in on 49 of the most highly regarded research findings in medicine over the previous 13 years, as judged by the science community's two standard measures: the papers had appeared in the journals most widely cited in research articles, and the 49 articles themselves were the most widely cited articles in these journals.....Ioannidis was putting his contentions to the test not against run-of-the-mill research, or even merely well-accepted research, but against the absolute tip of the research pyramid. **Of the 49 articles, 45 claimed to have uncovered effective interventions. Thirty-four of these claims had been retested, and 14 of these, or 41%, had been convincingly shown to be wrong or significantly exaggerated.** If between a third and a half of the most acclaimed research in medicine was proving untrustworthy, the scope and impact of the problem were undeniable. That article was published in the *Journal of the American Medical Association*.

On the relatively rare occasions when a study does go on long enough to track mortality, the findings frequently upend those of the shorter studies. (For example, though the vast majority of studies of overweight individuals link excess weight to ill health, the longest of them haven't convincingly shown that overweight people are likely to die sooner, and a few of them have seemingly demonstrated that moderately overweight people are likely to live longer.)

And so it goes for all medical studies, he says. Indeed, nutritional studies aren't the worst. Drug studies have the added corruptive force of financial conflict of interest. The exciting links between genes and various diseases and traits that are relentlessly hyped in the press for heralding miraculous around-the-corner treatments for everything from colon cancer to schizophrenia have in the past proved so vulnerable to error and distortion, Ioannidis has found, that in some cases you'd have done about as well by throwing darts at a chart of the genome. (These studies seem to have improved somewhat in recent years, but whether they will hold up or be useful in treatment are still open questions.) Vioxx, Zelnorm, and Baycol were among the widely prescribed drugs found to be safe and effective in large randomized controlled trials before the drugs were yanked from the market as unsafe or not so effective, or both.

"Often the claims made by studies are so extravagant that you can immediately cross them out without needing to know much about the specific problems with the studies," Ioannidis says...."**Even when the evidence shows that a particular research idea is wrong, if you have thousands of scientists who have invested their careers in it, they'll continue to publish papers on it. It's like an epidemic, in the sense that they're infected with these wrong ideas, and they're spreading it to other researchers through journals.**"

Though scientists and science journalists are constantly talking up the value of the peer-review process, researchers admit among themselves that biased, erroneous, and even blatantly fraudulent studies easily slip through it. *Nature*, the grande dame of science journals, stated in a 2006 Editorial, "Scientists understand that peer-review per se provides only a minimal assurance of quality, and that the public conception of peer-review as a stamp of authentication is far from the truth." **What's more, the peer-review process often pressures researchers to shy away from striking out in genuinely new directions, and instead to build on the findings of their colleagues** (that is, their potential reviewers) in ways that only seem like breakthroughs — as with the exciting-sounding gene linkages (autism genes identified!) and nutritional findings (olive oil lowers blood pressure!) that are really just dubious and conflicting variations on a theme.

Most journal editors don't even claim to protect against the problems that plague these studies. University and government research overseers rarely step in to directly enforce research quality, and when they do, the science community goes ballistic over the outside interference. The ultimate protection against research error and bias is supposed to come from the way scientists constantly retest each other's results — except they don't....Of those 45 super-cited studies that Ioannidis focused on, 11 had never been retested. **Perhaps worse, Ioannidis found that even when a research error is outed, it typically persists for years or even decades.** He looked at three prominent health studies from the 1980s and 1990s that were each later soundly refuted, and discovered that researchers continued to cite the original results as correct more often than as flawed — in one case for at least 12 years after the results were discredited.

Doctors may notice that their patients don't seem to fare as well with certain treatments as the literature would lead them to expect, but the field is appropriately conditioned to subjugate such anecdotal evidence to study findings. Yet much, perhaps even most, of what doctors do has never been formally put to the test in credible studies, given that the need to do so became obvious to the field only in the 1990s, leaving it playing catch-up with a century or more of non-evidence-based medicine, and contributing to Ioannidis's shockingly high estimate of the degree to which medical knowledge is flawed. That we're not routinely made seriously ill by this shortfall, he argues, is due largely to the fact that most medical interventions and advice don't address life-and-death situations, but rather aim to leave us marginally healthier or less unhealthy, so we usually neither gain nor risk all that much.

But we expect more of scientists, and especially of medical scientists, given that we believe we are staking our lives on their results. The public hardly recognizes how bad a bet this is. The medical community itself might still be largely oblivious to the scope of the problem, if Ioannidis hadn't forced a confrontation when he published his studies in 2005.

But his bigger worry, he says, is that while his fellow researchers seem to be getting the message, he hasn't necessarily forced anyone to do a better job. He fears he won't in the end have done much to improve anyone's health. "There may not be fierce objections to what I'm saying," he explains. "But it's difficult to change the way that everyday doctors, patients, and healthy people think and behave."....It's not that he envisions doctors making all their decisions based solely on solid evidence — there's simply too much complexity in patient treatment to pin down every situation with a great study. **"Doctors need to rely on instinct and judgment to make choices,"** **he says. "But these choices should be as informed as possible by the** **evidence. And if the evidence isn't good, doctors should know that, too.** **And so should patients....**If we don't tell the public about these problems, then we're no better than nonscientists who falsely claim they can heal," he says. "If the drugs don't work and we're not sure how to treat something, why should we claim differently?

We could solve much of the wrongness problem, Ioannidis says, if the world simply stopped expecting scientists to be right. That's because being wrong in science is fine, and even necessary — as long as scientists recognize that they blew it, report their mistake openly instead of disguising it as a success, and then move on to the next thing, until they come up with the very occasional genuine breakthrough. **But as long as careers remain contingent on producing a stream of research that's dressed up to seem more right than it is, scientists will keep delivering exactly that.**

"Science is a noble endeavor, but it's also a low-yield endeavor," he says. "I'm not sure that more than a very small percentage of medical research is ever likely to lead to major improvements in clinical outcomes and quality of life. We should be very comfortable with that fact."

David H. Freedman is also the author of the book *Wrong: Why Experts Keep Failing Us — And How to Know When Not to Trust Them*. Here are some quotations from that book, as they appeared in the June 10, 2010 issue of *Atlantic Magazine*.

"A good doctor, it is presumed, scans the journals for the results of these studies to see what works and what doesn't on which patients, and how well and with what risks, modifying her practices accordingly. Does it make sense to prescribe an antibiotic to a child with an ear infection? Should middle-aged men with no signs of heart disease be told to take a small, daily dose of aspirin? Do the potential benefits of a particular surgical intervention outweigh the risks? Studies presumably provide the answers. In examining hundreds of these studies, **Dr. Ioannidis did indeed spot a pattern — a disturbing one. When a study was published, often it was only a matter of months, and at most a few years, before other studies came out to either fully refute the findings or declare that the results were "exaggerated"** in the sense that later papers revealed significantly lesser benefits to the treatment under study. Results that held up were outweighed two-to-one by results destined to be labeled "never mind."

What was going on here? The whole point of carrying out a study was to rigorously examine a question using tools and techniques that would yield solid data, allowing a careful and conclusive analysis that would replace the conjecture, assumptions, and sloppy assessments that had preceded it. The data were supposed to be the path to truth. And yet these studies, and most types of studies Ioannidis looked at, were far more often than not driving to wrong answers. They exhibited the sort of wrongness rate you would associate more with fad-diet tips, celebrity gossip, or political punditry than with state-of-the-art medical research.

The two-out-of-three wrongness rate Ioannidis found is worse than it sounds. He had been examining only the less than one-tenth of one percent of published medical research that makes it to the most prestigious medical journals. In other words, in determining that two-thirds of published medical research is wrong, Ioannidis is offering what can easily be seen as an extremely optimistic assessment. Throw in the presumably less careful work from lesser journals, and take into account the way the results end up being spun and misinterpreted by university and industrial PR departments and by journalists, and it's clear that whatever it was about expert wrongness that Ioannidis had stumbled on in these journals, the wrongness rate would only worsen from there.

Ioannidis felt he was confronting a mystery that spoke to the very foundation of medical wisdom. How can the research community claim to know what it's doing, and to be making significant progress, if it can't bring out studies in its top journals that correctly prove anything, or lead to better patient care?...**Nor did the problems appear to be unique to medicine: looking at other branches of science, including chemistry, physics, and psychology, he found much the same. "The facts suggest that for many, if not the majority, of fields, the majority of published studies are likely to be wrong," he says. Probably, he adds, "the vast majority."**

Putting trust in experts who are probably wrong is only part of the problem....So what if experts are usually wrong? That's the nature of expert knowledge — it progresses slowly as it feels its way through difficult questions. Well, sure, we live in a complex world without easy answers, so we might well expect to see our experts make plenty of missteps as they steadily chip away at the truth. I'm not saying that experts don't make any progress, or that they ought to have figured it all out long ago. I'm suggesting three things:

- We ought to be fully aware of how large a percentage of expert advice is flawed; we should find out if there are perhaps much more disconcerting reasons why experts so frequently get off track other than "that's just the nature of the beast"
- We ought to take the trouble to see if we can come up with clues that will help distinguish better expert advice from fishier stuff.
- And, by the way, if experts are so comfortable with the notion that their efforts ought to be expected to spit out mostly wrong answers, why don't they work a little harder to get this useful piece of information across to us when they're interviewed on morning news shows or in newspaper articles, and not just when they're confronted with their errors?

What About the Media?

In his January 2, 2013 *Atlantic Magazine* article, *Survival of the wrongest*, David H. Freedman discusses how personal-health journalism ignores the fundamental pitfalls baked into all scientific research and serves up a daily diet of unreliable information. Here are some direct quotes from that article.

"In all areas of personal health, we see prominent media reports that directly oppose well-established knowledge in the field, or that make it sound as if scientifically unresolved questions have been resolved. The media, for instance, have variously supported and shot down the notion that vitamin D supplements can protect against cancer, and that taking daily and low doses of aspirin extends life by protecting against heart attacks. Some reports have argued that frequent consumption of even modest amounts of alcohol leads to serious health risks, while others have reported that daily moderate alcohol consumption can be a healthy substitute for exercise. Articles sang the praises of new drugs like Avastin and Avandia before other articles deemed them dangerous, ineffective, or both.

What's going on? The problem is not, as many would reflexively assume, the sloppiness of poorly trained science writers looking for sensational headlines, and ignoring scientific evidence in the process. Many of these articles were written by celebrated health-science journalists and published in respected magazines and newspapers; their arguments were backed up with what appears to be solid, balanced reporting and the careful citing of published scientific findings.

But personal-health journalists have fallen into a trap. Even while following what are considered the guidelines of good science reporting, they still manage to write articles that grossly mislead the public, often in ways that can lead to poor health decisions with catastrophic consequences. Blame a combination of the special nature of health advice, serious challenges in medical research, and the failure of science journalism to scrutinize the research it covers.

...Gary Schwitzer, a former University of Minnesota journalism researcher and now publisher of health care-journalism watchdog HealthNewsReview.org,...conducted a study in 2008 of 500 health-related stories published over a 22-month period in large newspapers. The results suggested that not only has personal-health coverage become invasively and inappropriately ubiquitous, it is of generally questionable quality, with about two-thirds of the articles found to have major flaws. **The errors** included **exaggerating the prevalence and ravages of a disorder, ignoring potential side effects and other downsides to treatments, and failing to discuss alternative treatment options.** In the survey, 44% of the 256 staff journalists who responded said that their organizations at times base stories almost entirely on press releases.

When science journalism goes astray, the usual suspect is a failure to report accurately and thoroughly on research published in peer-reviewed journals....the findings of published studies are beset by a number of problems that tend to make them untrustworthy, or at least render them exaggerated or oversimplified....Biostatisticians have studied the question of just how frequently published studies come up with wrong answers. **A highly regarded researcher in this subfield of medical wrongness is John Ioannidis, who heads the Stanford Prevention Research Center,....[he] has determined that the overall wrongness rate in medicine's top journals is about two thirds, and that estimate has been well-accepted in the medical field.**

Another frequent claim, especially within science journalism, is that the wrongness problems go away when reporters stick with randomized control trials (RCTs)....**Ioannidis and others have found that RCTs, too (even large ones), are plagued with inaccurate findings, if to a lesser extent. Remember that virtually every drug that gets pulled off the market when dangerous side effects emerge was proven safe in a large RCT.**

Why do studies end up with wrong findings?...To cite just a few of these problems:

- **Mismeasurement – To test the safety and efficacy of a drug,...**scientists must rely on animal studies, <u>which tend to translate poorly to humans</u>, and on various short-cuts and indirect measurements in human studies that they hope give them a good indication of what a new drug is doing. The difficulty of setting up good human studies, and of making relevant, accurate measurements on people, plagues virtually all medical research.
- **Confounders – Study subjects may lose weight on a certain diet, but was it because of the diet, or because of the support they got from doctors and others running the study?**
- **Publication bias – Research journals, like newsstand magazines, want exciting stories that will have impact on readers.** That means they prefer studies that deliver the most interesting and important findings....since scientists' careers depend on being published in prominent journals, and because

there is intense competition to be published, scientists much prefer to come up with the exciting, important findings journals are looking for — even if its a wrong finding....A reporter who accurately reports findings is probably transmitting wrong findings.

It's not nearly enough to include in news reports the few mild qualifications attached to any study (the study wasn't large, the effect was modest, some subjects withdrew from the study partway through it). **Readers ought to be alerted, as a matter of course, to the fact that wrongness is embedded in the entire research system, and that few medical research findings ought to be considered completely reliable, regardless of the type of study, who conducted it, where it was published, or who says its a good study.**

When a reporter, for whatever reasons, wants to demonstrate that a particular type of diet works better than others or that diets never work, there is a wealth of studies that will back him or her up, never mind all those other studies that have found exactly the opposite (or the studies can be mentioned, then explained away as flawed)....**Questioning most health-related findings isn't denying good science; its demanding it.**

Yet in health journalism (and in science journalism in general), scientists are treated as trustworthy heroes, and journalists proudly brag on their websites about the awards and recognition they've received from science associations, as if our goal should be to win the admiration of the scientists we're covering, and to make it clear we're eager to return the favor....given what we know about the problems with scientific studies, anyone who wants to assert that science is being carried out by an army of Abraham Lincolns has a lot of explaining to do. Scientists themselves don't make such a claim, so why would we do it on their behalf? We owe readers more than that. Their lives may depend on it."

1 Your Health is Your Responsibility

My main objective is to make you think. Don't just look at the propaganda; don't just look at the salespeople or the advertising; 95% of what I see on television today is unbelievable. It is there to sell the product and has nothing to do with the quality of the product. This is especially true in the food field. Stay away from it.

Life to me is like a three-legged stool. As long as the three legs are in balance, the top of your stool is perfectly horizontal; therefore, you don't have any problems. But if one leg gets a little bit shorter than the other two, the top of your stool is going to turn off to the side. That becomes your problem of life because you constantly keep sliding off the stool.

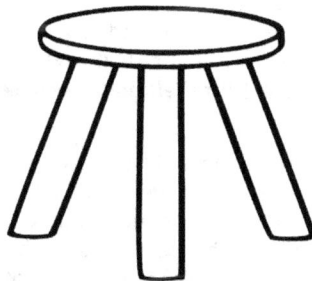

What do these three legs stand for? They stand for the intellectual, the spiritual and the physical. So you see, you have to fortify each a little every day to make sure you can solve your problems and stay on a horizontal plane. Remember that at all times.

My father taught me as a youth that, if I had not learned one new thing each day, that day was wasted and would never come back. The other thing he said to me was, "Son, no matter how stupid an individual is, he knows one thing that you do not know, and it pays you to listen to it." Another thing that my father used to say was, "When you're green, you grow; when you're ripe, you rot!" Think about that one.

Editor: At the time Dr. Ellis made these statements to his audience (1985), he had just appeared on Ed Busch's syndicated America Overnight radio show. He received over 370 letters and 111 telephone calls as a result of his appearance. This response was astounding, as the show was only two hours long, beginning at midnight.

Take Charge of Your Health

It is vitally important for each thinking adult to inform himself with respect to how he should live, what habits he should retain, and which ones he shall discard. Many of the simplest habits, such as smoking and drinking alcohol, are just as harmful as the vicious or immoral ones! Eating sweet rolls and drinking tea can get you into trouble just as certainly as alcohol and tobacco.

What has nature designed for you as a plan for healthy living? Do you have any idea? Well, carry on reading! Poor health is primarily a result of poor eating (nutritional) habits. **You, and only you, have the power of decision regarding what foods you eat; therefore, the choice is up to you!** As my father used to say, **"Regardless how bad any situation is, if you want to be truly honest with yourself, you can always find out where you were at fault!" Such is a wonderful revelation, because it is the first step in taking charge.**

If you are seriously interested in making the desired corrections, they are within your capabilities, because a wealth of information is now available concerning diet and nutrition. **However, a doctor is only as good as the cooperation he receives from his patient; so, when you start a program, stick with it long enough to get results.** Do not allow yourself to get discouraged! Often, when the body starts to change from the diseased state to the healthy state, reactions will take place that may make you feel like the cure is worse than the disease. These reaction periods last for about 10 days, so simply prepare yourself for it, and be determined that you will keep working toward the worthwhile reward ahead! Consider these issues:

- Surgery can remove an organ or part after it is too badly diseased to function; but surgery cannot heal or replace the organ or part.
- Drugs may alleviate or remove the symptoms of a disease, but they cannot remove the cause of the disease.
- Manipulations will aid structural or body balance and restore a certain amount of circulation and nerve flow to the affected organ or part, but they cannot change the quality of the blood or nerve fluids that are flowing to that organ or part.
- The mind can alter one's attitude about life, but it cannot completely deal with the physical causes of disease. You must learn as much as you can about the natural laws before you can understand why only one or two techniques is not sufficient.

Holistic health takes a complete commitment, intelligent eating habits, proper sleep, proper attitude, and proper physical care. It is nothing less, and you cannot cheat the system by omitting any one of the above. You can only cheat yourself directly and your loved ones indirectly! You must be disciplined. If you're not willing to follow all of the rules and regulations set down by your health doctor, you're not going to get anywhere. After all, when you get sick, it is you who have allowed your body to deteriorate by not keeping it free of toxins and neglecting to give it the vitamins, minerals, enzymes, coenzymes, hormones, proteins, fats, and carbohydrates that it needs and deserves. Incidentally, have you been breathing clean air and drinking pure water?

Public Image of the Body

How does industry and, consequently, the general public envision the human body? They do so in terms of information that is part of commercial, so-called nutritional campaigns that give rise to food fads. Over the years, the calorie theory has had its rise to fame and its decline to oblivion. The vitamin principle, the chemical characterization of foods in an attempt to fit the food to the body by a detailed analysis of the assumed need at the time, has not worked either. Neither of the methods nor the assumptions upon which they were based successfully dealt with the problems of health; the people who were so analyzed were looking for a crutch. **None of the techniques restored health to the degree desired. Why? Because none of the theories took into account the fact the body is more than a crude chemical laboratory or furnace that simply burns up food for the human**

engine. The human body is much more complex than their systems analyses could handle.

Just because one may eat a product without dropping dead or immediately falling ill is no proof that the product is even a marginally suitable item for consumption. Most deficiencies do not appear for weeks, months, or, perhaps, years later — when the cause of the problem is long forgotten and ignored!

As you can see, our most difficult task is to fight the constant bombardment of the people with this ill-conceived media attack on the viewing and listening public. The sole interest of companies who advertise in this way is to sell products and maximize profits. As P. T. Barnum once said, "If you tell a lie big enough and often enough, the greatest majority of people will believe it." Drug trusts are stopping us from getting the truth. You know, all colleges today are subsidized by industry. If they get subsidized high enough, believe you me, they are going to teach what is in accordance to get that money from that industrial grant.

General Health Tips

To get started, below are listed tips for a healthier life. Some activities need to be developed without delay, while others can be incorporated over time, but only with sincere application on your part. Most of these are repeated and expanded upon in later portions of this book. For now, read them over and resolve to be open-minded. You may copy this list and share it with others.

1. Be aware of your health needs. Be aware of your disease possibilities like cavities in your teeth, sinusitis, infections, constipation, sores and cuts that do not heal rapidly, and being overweight.

2. Rest and relax according to your individual need. For some people, eight hours of sleep is sufficient; others need six. Some others need ten.

3. Form a regular bowel habit. If you are reducing in weight and working toward your normal weight, you should have two or three movements daily. Drink a full glass of water upon arising to strt peristalsis. Report irregularities such as constipation or excessively loose movements to a physician.

4. Breathe fresh air and get some sunlight, but not too much!

5. Enjoy life. We live today, on yesterday's experiences to make a better tomorrow.

6. See a health doctor who's interested in making you healthy; do not see a disease doctor who's only interested in relieving your symptoms. When you're at your doctor's office, look at him; does he look healthy? If he's healthy himself, he'll be able to teach you how to get healthy. But if he looks sick, or is big and fat, how can he tell you to reduce your weight or get your health back?

7. Get a health survey done at least once a year. This consists of your blood, hair, and urine analysis. Have your doctor check your blood chemistry levels of Total Protein, Albumin, and Globulin to see if you have sufficient hydrochloric acid (HCl) in your stomach to digest proteins and fats. There's no such condition as over acidity of he stomach. Today, bottle-fed babies start running out of sufficient HCl in their late teens and early twenties. Most everybody over 50 years old needs HCl supplements.

8. Follow the instructions about which foods and drinks to consume and to avoid, as shown in Specific Food Recommendations on page 57. Remember, if you eat junk foods, you will have a junky body. Eat health or natural foods, and you will be naturally healthy.

9. Read the book written by Jane Armstrong, *Pick your Poison*. Study what's in foods that you eat. Avoid all food containing artificial coloring. These dyes are highly cancer-causing.

10. The most important factors in your diet to get in balance are proteins, vitamins, and minerals. Vitamins are the catalysts that make the minerals become the enzymes. Protein is needed in every single function of the body. Vitamins and minerals must be in their proper balance and in ratio to one another, otherwise they will break down and not perform properly. This to me is the basic cause of disease.

11. Do not overcook protein with high temperature. Keep it on the rare side, and cook at an internal temperature of 138° F.

12. Be careful with salt. Have your doctor check your blood levels of sodium and potassium for proper balance. If not balanced, they destroy circulation and make you nervous. You may need to consume salt to maintain the balance; be absolutely sure about the levels in the blood before reducing salt intake.

13. Learn how to blend food so that you can eat it digestibly.

14. Eat foods that can spoil but eat them before they spoil.

15. Include adequate bulk type food such as bran, celery, lettuce, etc.

Your Health is Your Responsibility

16. Include food rich in B17 (the seeds of all fruit have it, with the exception of citrus seeds, especially peaches, pears, apples, and apricots.)

17. Do not eat food that you know produces gas.

18. Chew your foods thoroughly; they must be near liquid before swallowing.

19. Do not use aluminum cookware or aluminum foil on foods, as it has been found to devitalize food.

20. Drink at least 8-10 eight-ounce glasses of fluid daily. The body needs this amount to carry on all functions. you perspire an amount equal to the amount of urination per day. Avoid hot or excessively cold beverages.

21. Drink distilled water and supplement to your mineral deficiencies. Before drinking spring, well, or even city water, have it analyzed and checked with the health doctor to see if it's good to drink. Do not drink chlorinated water or ingest organic chlorides in any form, as they are now found to cause cancer and have also been found to destroy HCl formation in your stomach.

22. Exercise daily; it's a must for health. Walk or swim two miles a day or ride a bicycle 10 miles a day. That comes out of the International College of Fine Nutrition program.

23. Learn how to balance your body. Research has shown that 62% of the population has an anatomical short leg. The standing X-ray of the lumbar spine and pelvis is the method to ascertain which leg and how much. Use both a heel and sole lift for balance; do not build up only the heel.

24. Avoid using synthetic chemicals for your skin and hair, such as cosmetics, colognes, hair tints, and dyes. For ladies, don't wear bras and panty hose made from synthetic materials, but use cotton panties.

25. Do not smoke, keep away from the smoke of others. Second-hand smoke is worse than first-hand smoking, because you mix it with the carbon dioxide coming out of your breath, and it changes the chemistry of the nicotine and sulfuric acid from the paper.

26. Avoid chemicals in your environment, such as in paint and solvents used to clean tools.

27. Avoid all aerosol containers, such as found in insecticide, deodorant, and air fresheners.

28. If you have to wear dark glasses outside, get a full spectrum lens. Do not use fluorescent bulbs; use Spectrolights.

29. Avoid radiation from microwave towers, microwave ovens, and television sets (color is three times worse than black-and-white).

Break the Laws and Pay the Price

Many people make a serious mistake in assuming that their bodies are their own to do with as they desire. Our Creator lends bodies to individuals during their short stays on this earth, so that they may express themselves physically, emotionally, mentally, and spiritually. For this loan, like any other kind of loan, our Creator demands payment; but this payment, unlike any other financial obligation, is very reasonable. The payment consists of diligent care and nourishing of these bodies in full conformity to the terms and conditions as outlined by our Creator in the Holy Scriptures. These laws have been known throughout the ages as Natural Laws.

No man, no matter how hard he may try, can escape his vital relation to the universe, as it is forever fixed by these laws. These laws are absolutely non-yielding and are constantly and vigorously enforced by powers beyond any man's control. Remember, each time you break these laws, you must pay! There is no escape; there is no chance of not being caught! You will be penalized by worry, disease, fear, confusion, discontent, insecurity, anger, insanity, and a broken life; then you head for the underground bungalow.

You cannot go to a doctor and say, "I've broken all of the laws of God and nature, but I expect to get better because you're going to give me some miracle pills." It just doesn't work that way. Conformity to these laws always brings its own rewards. As proof of this statement, remember Proverbs 3:1-2 that says, "My son, forget not my law; but let thine heart keep my commandments. For length of days and long life and peace, shall they add to thee."

Your Health is Your Responsibility

2 Protein Nutrition

I don't want you to believe anything I tell you just because I say it. But before you condemn it, try it out over a long enough period of time to prove whether I'm right or wrong. That to me, is the key to understanding all of these concepts.

Just as a building is only as good as the weakest brick in its structure, the human body is only as strong as the weakest cell. You had better take care of every cell, and they are up in the trillions. It is estimated that your brain has 26 billion. So it is important that you think in terms of maintaining the total body — not Isolated parts. You have to maintain everything. You have to get the ingredients in that body and the bloodstream and, if you are a supporter of spinal manipulation, have a competent professional normalize the nerve supply to the organs and other systems.

Physiology and Diet

Today, every school student has the opportunity to learn, in the study of human physiology, that the cells of the body are constantly being rebuilt. Some parts of the body are renewed as often as once a month. Much of the body is renewed every year, but the bones of the skeleton require about seven years for their complete replacement. The bloodstream constantly brings fresh building material to every cell and carries away the waste products of metabolism. **The only way the body is able to rebuild itself is from the material carried to it by the bloodstream.** If any part lacks health and efficient function, it is because the material brought by the blood has been unsuitable for the task of maintaining healthy tissue. The only source from which the blood can derive these rebuilding materials is by absorption through the walls of the intestines of food substances that have been put into the digestive tract — ingested foods. Therefore, the fact that you are unhealthy shows that you have failed to put the proper substances into the digestive tract. **Unless you have been subjected to external injury, the lack of nutritional factors is the cause of your disease.**

Importance of Protein to Metabolism

How important are proteins? **Researchers at the University of Illinois Medical School have demonstrated that proteins are the most important substances in our diet.** Their report, published in the late 1940s, was of great interest to physicians who wanted to apply the principles stated therein to their patients.

It is the lack of available protein that causes one to get old! Sufficient protein containing all of the amino acids is required for body synthesis and producing protein tissues for repair and maintenance of muscle, hair, fingernails, heart, brain, and all vital organs, in addition to enzymes and hormones secreted by the ductless glands. Indeed, without utilizable protein, there is no life. There is no disease, illness, or abnormality in the body that is not, in some way, related to protein metabolism.

- There are protein molecules in the bloodstream (albumin and globulin are two) that are carriers for other materials such as enzymes, minerals, fats, sugars, vitamins, and hormones.
- Enzymes and many hormones are themselves protein in nature.
- The red blood cells are mainly protein, the oxygen-carrying component, hemoglobin, being a globular protein.
- All of the endocrine glands unite molecules of proteins with molecules of other substances to form hormones. For example, thyroid protein plus iodine equals thyroxine, pancreas protein plus zinc equals insulin.
- Through the action of proteolytic enzymes and vitamin and mineral catalysts, proteins are broken down into amino acids. These are absorbed and assimilated through the intestinal wall and carried through the portal circulation to the liver.
  Two of the 10 essential amino acids, arginine and histidine, are vital to growing youngsters. The body uses 26 amino acids, and 16 of these can be synthesized in the liver, primarily from the 10 essential ones. Methionine, another essential amino acid, is a precursor to the important lipotropic factors, choline and inositol. Interestingly, all of the essential amino acids must be present in the body and in sufficient quantity at the same time.

Otherwise, the nutritional effectiveness of the entire group is impaired.

Proteins are not stored in the body in the form in which they are ingested. The assimilated amino acids are transformed into storage proteins, the predominant one being albumin. This albumin is the internal source of amino acids; the diet is the external source. However, the amino acids will not be utilized unless there is a normal complement in the body of gonadal or sex hormones. Adults tend to expend protein excessively. Business and social pressures, insufficient rest, pregnancy, and lactation all cost more protein than most of us can spare. The body that doesn't have a regular dietary supply of protein must steal protein from wherever it can to keep going. Any cell might be robbed. The joints are the first to be looted. As the body uses more proteins and if the stored supply is inadequate, they may be taken from any tissue, even though the tissues involved may not be able to spare any of their own protoplasmic proteins.

At the stage of senility, lack of steroids from the adrenal cortex may be a cause of protein deficiencies. In many arthritics, there is anemia, secondary in nature with all evidences of inflammation − characteristic of usage of proteins at an accelerated rate. A patient with a high fever uses proteins more rapidly and presents a greater hypoproteinemia than one who may not be eating enough proteins. **In arthritis or bursitis, the body will make an effort to maintain serum albumin (storage protein) levels by taking protoplasmic albumin from the joint surfaces themselves. The more taken, the more severe is trauma to the joints.** Cortisone or ACTH, by releasing albumin from the muscle tissues, makes it available to the blood and thus to the joint surfaces, decreasing the irritability and inflammation − the arthritic manifestations in the joints. However, as you notice, this is done at the expense of the muscle tissue! This leads to protein depletion in other tissues even though the arthritic symptoms have been relieved. Remember that, for a gram of protein available in the bloodstream, the healthy joint surface requires 30 times as much.

When protein intake equals protein usage, a balance exists and is expressed in terms of nitrogen balance. If more protein is used than is replaced by ingestion and assimilation, a negative nitrogen balance exists. **An excellent criterion of protein availability to the tissues is the state of the skin, hair, and fingernails. Coarse, brittle hair that falls out easily; dry, hard skin that wrinkles easily or is not elastic; and fingernails that crack, split or do not grow properly are all indications of inavailability of proteins.** This inavailability of sufficient amounts of protein can be caused by inefficient intake in the diet, poor mastication, poor digestion, poor absorption, poor assimilation (aberrant enzyme, vitamin, and mineral metabolism), and improper levels of the sex hormones. Other signs of protein deficiency are fatigue, sensitivity to cold, evident pallor, allergies, most edema, hypertension, and a negative attitude. In fact, children who are highly nervous, irritating, defiant, and mischievous are those children who are eating large amounts of sugars and starches. They eat very little protein-rich foods!

Quoting from the article, *Arthritis Isn't Hopeless to This Doctor*, *Prevention* magazine, July 1968, interview with Dr. Ellis, "...especially among older people, **proteins go through the system largely undigested. But the human body is such that, at any cost, it will keep the blood supply of protein (albumin) constant and adequate. If the protein does not come from the blood, the body will draw it out of the tissues. If the protein is taken from the bursas, the collagen will break down and bursitis will develop. If from the tendons, tendosynovitis will result. If from the joints, arthritis; if from the muscles, rheumatism.**

The water supply in most of our major cities hasn't helped the situation any. For example, the pH of Pittsburgh's drinking water, which should be around 7, was 8.2 a few years ago. Now it is 8.8. They pour alkalai (calcium and magnesium carbonate (lime), sodium hydroxide, aluminum sulfate (alum), iron chloride) into the reservoir to encourage coagulation and flocculation to reduce dirt and bacteria. But these same alkalies raise the likelihood of painful arthritis."

Dr. Ellis' Own Physical Breakdown

The reason why I learned so much about digestion and assimilation of food was because I had a physical breakdown at age 29. I found out that I had no production of hydrochloric acid in my stomach at all — absolutely none. At that time, I made my own hydrochloric acid. I had to carry it in a glass-stoppered bottle with a glass straw and dropper everywhere I went. I would get an eight-ounce glass of water, pull out the bottle, and put 10 drops into the glass. When I wanted to drink it, I would use the straw and have to curl my tongue and suck it up because if it hit my teeth, it would dissolve them.

Today we have betaine hydrochloride tablets. Also, we are lucky to have protein supplements in the form available today. When I started out trying to get a protein supplement, we didn't have them on the market. We had to drink raw meat drippings.

Protein Intake

First, we must eat a variety of protein sources animal and vegetable. When we tell a patient that he is deficient in proteins, he will usually say, "But doctor, I eat plenty of meat or protein food!" This shows how necessary it is to know the difference between eating sufficient amounts of protein foods and eating sufficient amounts of protein foods that contain the essential amino acids in the proper ratios!

Are you getting enough protein? One way to determine this is to multiply your weight by two to get the number of protein calories required per day. The best animal proteins are turkey, lamb, beef, fish, fowl, eggs, and gelatin (lacks tryptophan).

Protein Digestion

The first step in halting protein thievery is to have ample protein in the diet. But, it is equally true that the richest protein diet won't prevent a degenerative disease if the protein is poorly assimilated by the system. What is the next step necessary to ensure that these proteins become available for use by our bodies? Digestion! Let's start at the beginning and work into the needs and problems. First, we must masticate our proteins as we do all food in our mouth to break up the large pieces, mix them with saliva, and thereby prepare them for the other digestive processes to follow.

It is in the stomach that our greatest, and consequently our most serious problem exists. This problem is the widespread lack in our population of gastric digestive power in the form of hydrochloric acid and pepsin. Also essential are inositol, choline, methionine, trypsin, and chymotrypsin. Pepsin, the only digestive enzyme present in the adult stomach, is the stimulator for the production of hydrochloric acid. In fact, peppermint is a stimulator of pepsin production; peppermint tea is beneficial with meals to induce acid production. Acidity is needed to activate the peristaltic wave and open the pyloric valve of the stomach; it also stimulates the emptying of bile from the liver and gallbladder. When the stomach is too alkaline, and fermentation or putrefaction takes place, the gallbladder is falsely triggered, bile is regurgitated back into the stomach, and a burning sensation is experienced (heartburn). People who have an acetone smell on their breath are not digesting their food. The starches and sugars ferment; fats and proteins putrefy. You can tell the difference in that the fermentation gives a breath similar to that of alcoholism. The putrefaction gives a really foul breath. With sufficient stomach acid, the digestion will be complete, and there will be no odors.

There are several methods of determining whether we have an adequate supply of gastric secretions. One may swallow a small collection tube after a test breakfast and directly measure the hydrochloric acid content of the measured volume. A newer test is called Diagnex Blue. This test is conducted by swallowing a couple of these pills and measuring the dye as it is excreted in the urine in a given period of time. **How does a lack of hydrochloric acid manifest itself? Symptoms are a lack of appetite, distaste for meat, burping, a sense of fullness an hour or two after eating, and a burning or itching rectum.**

Scientists have shown that the maximum production of hydrochloric acid is reached in persons of age 25; by the age of 40, it has diminished by 15%. By the age of 65, the production has diminished by 85%. The point is that, the older you get, the less able you are to digest proteins properly.

Remember what I said about advertising on TV, radio, and in magazines? Those companies who propagate such advertising claims would have you believe that everyone is over acidic and that everyone needs antacid tablets! Nothing could be further from the truth! Did you know that the symptoms of an over-acid stomach are exactly the same as those of an alkaline stomach? **With the lack of acid, bile backs up into the stomach, the highly alkaline bile irritates the stomach lining, and a burning develops.**

Why not try a simple test to see if this assumption is correct? The next time you have a full feeling in the stomach, a burning sensation, or if you are burping, take a teaspoon of apple cider vinegar in a small amount of water. You will be surprised how quickly you will feel better! However, if the burning sensation increases, your stomach is truly over-acidic; this is not a common occurrence.

Protein Assimilation

Assimilation is the next important step in protein utilization by the body, and it depends on several factors. We must have adequate vitamins and minerals, especially vitamin C. In this case, vitamin C should include all components of the complex — civatemic acid, ascorbic acid, and bioflavonoids or vitamin P. It is of utmost importance to eat enough raw greens and fresh fruit to get this vitamin C or to take a complete supplement. With the proper balance of vitamins, minerals, and sex hormones, the proteins will be made assimilative. Remember, however, that the sex glands are the only glands that do not continue to function during your entire life. After castration by surgery, after the female menopause, or after the male climacteric, the sex organs cannot contribute to the endocrine balance of the body. If transfer of these duties from the sex glands to the adrenal glands or liver does not take place, a reaction occurs. This is called hot flashes in women and a loss of sex drive and great fatigue in men. Thymus, adrenal, and thyroid tissue are needed.

We must be able to absorb nutrients efficiently. Even when the sex glands are functioning very nicely, we can still inhibit protein assimilation by coating the lining of the stomach and intestinal membranes with mucous. **The most severe, mucous-forming food is milk, and this, I feel is the most notorious cause of malabsorption of nutrients. Suffice to say at this point, even though we eat a high protein diet and have the proper digestive enzyme, vitamins, minerals, and hormonal balance, we can defeat the purpose of protein ingestion by using milk products.** We must have a clean, unclogged bowel wall for the proper absorption and utilization of nutrients. Preservatives, such as potassium nitrate, can have serious effects on the glandular system. I have seen this in my own practice.

Allergic Responses to Protein

Proteins come from external sources such as meat, fish, eggs, fowl, and gelatin in one group. Nuts, seeds, and cereals constitute a separate group. A major consideration is the digestibility of them.

From the *Organic Consumer's Report* comes this statement, "Hay fever, asthma, and migraines are related to the body's inability to properly break proteins down completely into amino acids, preparing them to be used as building blocks to repair tissue, etc. This faulty process results in the buildup of uric acid and other toxins. Undigested proteins find their way into the bloodstream, setting up allergic reactions. The usual medical way of treating these allergies is to isolate individual allergens. This method usually involves a restricted diet and often causes the affected person to rely upon drugs to counteract the attacks."

Editor: See Clin Exp Immunol. 2008 Sep; 153(Suppl 1): 3-6, titled Allergy and the Gastrointestinal System, G Vighi, F Marcucci, L Sensi, G Di Cara, and F Frati.

Acid-Alkaline Balance

There is some misunderstanding about whether a food is acidic or alkaline and what it does to the body's (blood) pH. The blood pH remains very close to 7.4 (alkaline) regardless of what foods are consumed. However, we are concerned with the effect that eating certain foods or drinking certain beverages have on the pH of the urine. **If a food increases the acidity (lowers the pH) of the urine after it is ingested, it is classified as an acid-forming food. If a food increases the alkalinity (raises the pH) of the urine after it has been ingested, it is classified it as an alkaline-forming food.**

The acid-alkaline balance is of utmost importance in protein digestion and synthesis, yet it is often overlooked. **A diet high in protein produces residue that raises urine pH, increasing the chance of forming kidney and bladder stones.** Knowing his or her urine pH helps the individual adjust the diet to lower the pH of the kidneys and bladder. Care must be taken to avoid other alkaline-forming foods such as orange juice, which is highly acidic in the glass, but causes the urine to become alkaline. Others include tomato, and pineapple, with sweet milk running a close second. See Directions for Combining Foods on page 73.

Testing Urine pH

To determine urine pH, you can use a simple do-it-yourself test, using a small piece of chemically-treated testing paper (litmus or nitrozine). **Test the first urine voided upon arising or the first urine voided after breakfast. Both should be acid, pH 5.5 or 6 (below 7 is acid, 7.0 is neutral, and above 7 is alkaline). The second test is more important, for it is normal to be most acid about 4:00 AM.**

Restoring Urine Acidity

When the morning urine test indicates over-alkalinity (above pH 7), there are some reliable ways to return the pH of the bladder to acid.

- Follow the advice of Dr. Jarvis' in his book, *Folk Medicine*, which is to take two teaspoons of apple cider vinegar with a little honey in either hot or cold water.
- Another method is to use Digestin, one of the many hydrochloric acid tablet products available in health food stores, at each meal. The Digestin-type of digestive aid is a very good one, made from a combination of betaine HCl from beets, glutamic HCl from grains, plus small amounts of pepsin, bile, and often papain and vitamin B6. Consistent testing will help determine the amount needed by each person, as it is an individual problem.
- Consume bacteria as found in acidophilus or lactic acid fermenting yeast tablets.

- Consume cold processed, unsaturated vegetable oils with a high linoleic acid content. One example of the use of oil is described by Dr. Jarvis. It follows the results from the use of one tablespoon of corn oil at each meal (we don't want anybody using corn oil today, as it is sprayed 34 times in its growth process). Sesame and safflower oils are also high in linoleic acid, which when present, insures the synthesis of other valuable fatty acids such as linolenic, and oleic acid.

Walter B. Guy, M.D., prolific researcher in digestion and mineral utilization in the 1930s, attributed over-alkalinity and the resulting infiltration of the salts of urea into the lymph channels to be directly related to arthritis, diseased hearts, kidneys, and swollen joints. Hydrochloric acid is the only acid normally present in human tissue. When deficient, lactic acid, a waste by-product of muscular activity, increases. In the course of elimination, this is broken down to carbon dioxide, to be expelled by respiration, and glycogen, to be retained as tissue food.

Protein Nutrition

3 Food and Diet

> "If the doctor of today does not become the dietician of tomorrow, the dietician of today will become the doctor of tomorrow." - Dr. Alexio Carrell, Rockefeller Institute of Medical Research

Benjamin Franklin once wrote, "Would'st thou enjoy a long life, a healthy body, and a vigorous mind, and be acquainted with the wonderful works of God, labor in the first place to bring thy appetite to reason."

What you eat and how you eat it is what you are! You eat for health or you eat for disease; there is no in-between! If you do not buy wholesome food, you are on a disease diet. If you do not prepare it properly, you are on a disease diet. If you do not combine the foods properly, with respect to foods that are eaten at the same time, you are on a disease diet. Furthermore, if you overcook your food, you are on a disease diet. **Are you eating a disease diet?**

Today, as we are living in a chemical world, we have to change our diet to modern standards. We can no longer buy top quality foods (except those that are organically grown); instead, we are forced to accept foods raised for quantity with chemical fertilizers, fungicides, and bactericides. These same foods may be fortified or enriched, while others are processed, medicated, hormonized, pasteurized, degerminated, refined, hydrogenated, hardened, bleached, or what have you!

These processes — additions and subtractions to foods — are used as propaganda to entice the unsuspecting customer to buy and consume these products as being improved upon from the original. Unfortunately, the customer learns too late that this propaganda is not the truth, for, when they have been afflicted with disease, they learn, if they are fortunate enough to be taught, the bitter truth that is the basis of their problems!

Food and Diet

The following information is presented so that patients and their physicians can understand the principles of good diet as they relate to their own health. Patients should learn these principles so they can discipline themselves and have an appreciation for what their physician is doing to try to help them. Mutual cooperation is essential.

Physicians should think of what is to follow as valuable personally and professionally. Unless a physician understands the eating habits of patients and makes an effort to modify their undesirable eating habits, he or she cannot successfully treat these patients. Physicians must make it their business to discover these eating indiscretions; one good way to accomplish this is through a 7-Day Diet Journal. When a comprehensive profile is done for a patient, this journal is a necessary part. It is a very simple, but effective, information gathering tool. Just have the patient write down everything he or she eats for a period of seven days.

Editor: At the end of Dr. Ellis' career, he became aware of research involving tests for food, preservative, and coloring intolerances (not allergies) being carried out in San Antonio, Texas and Miami, Florida. He was hopeful that he would be able to incorporate such testing into his comprehensive plan, but the field was not commercialized by the time Dr. Ellis began his struggle with a terminal illness.

Subsequent to Dr. Ellis' passing, researchers developed what is called the ALCAT test and made it available to the public. Current information about this service is found at https://cellsciencesystems.com/patients/alcat-test/. An informative book about food intolerance and weight control is *Your Hidden Food Allergies Are Making You Fat* by Roger Deutsch and Rudy Rivera M.D., July 23, 2002, available from Amazon.com.

For a list of undesirable food additives, visit the MPH website at http://mphprogramslist.com/50-jawdroppingly-toxic-food-additives-to-avoid/.

Vegetarianism

I don't believe in vegetarianism. I have done over 2,000 blood, hair, and urine analyses on vegetarians. They all have very poor immune systems, and they are always anemic. We see problems as a result of these two factors. So many of these people look like they are a fugitive from a square meal.

In the Bible, there are 233 verses that tell you about eating meat; 83 tell you to eat beef, 61 to eat fish, and six to eat venison; but there's not a single verse that I can find that tells you to be a vegetarian.

Diet vs. Personality

What you eat affects your personality and emotions. Massachusetts Institute of Technology researcher, Dr. Richard Workman, says, "A lack of protein may lead to withdrawal and indifference. Too much sugar makes a person an emotional yo-yo; oversensitive, irrational, and jumpy." When you talk about sugar, the normal yearly consumption of sugar per person is five pounds. In the U.S. last year, the consumption was 140 pounds. The sugar content of most of today's childrens' cereals ranges from five to 55%. Any wonder that there are so many hyperkinetic children today? Not counting the 3,000 additives that Dr. Ben Feingold talks so much about. **The American Diabetic Society years ago made the statement that if the U.S. population continued to eat the amount of processed starches and sugars that they are now doing, everybody in the U.S. will be diabetic within 10 years!** It is very important to eat natural food in its natural state.

When you consider those factors of hypoglycemia, the forerunner of diabetes, figure how many of you with those symptoms and the direction that you're heading if you don't change your diet. Honey is among the best, but take it sparingly. Honey is made up of slow-absorbing sugars, whereas white sugar is a fast-absorbing sugar that overstimulates the pancreas. There's a great push of energy, but then insulin production goes too long and produces hypoglycemia. You get tired and useless again.

Even in the case of diabetes, you can use as much as two tablespoons a day of good blackstrap molasses. The mineral content of the molasses will help to stimulate the activity of developing insulin. You want to remember that insulin is manufactured in the beta cells of the Islets of Langerhans from zinc, chromium, and albumin (that is the part of the protein), and you also have to consider potassium because of what it does to the sugar metabolism within the liver.

Recommended Eating Habits

To ensure the success of this program, a patient must cooperate. Doctors should make sure that the patient keeps in contact with his or her office so that the patient can stay motivated and modifications to the program may be made as necessary.

The following are more instructions.

- **Establish a health diet.** Too often, people decrease their food intake to the point of decreasing metabolism. It is important that you have a normal daily intake of nutritious food. By establishing this habit you will find that you actually eat less and feel better for it! The menus listed below are not to be followed letter by letter, but they are considered to be a pattern of eating by which it is possible for you to achieve a correct balance of carbohydrates, proteins, and fats.
- **Choose your foods wisely.** Taste and hunger should not be the sole reason for food choice, but these foods can be appealing as to appearance and taste. Keep on a high protein, low fat, low calorie diet. This means emphasizing the protein foods such as meat, eggs, fish, fowl, whole grains, and gelatin.

  It is my opinion that it is best for us to eat as many organically raised foods as possible to obtain the highest quality. If prepared properly and eaten slowly with thorough mastication to assure a proper start in digestion, the foods can supply us with the nutrients we need for better health. As Charles F. Kettering said, "We should all be concerned about the future because we will have to spend the rest of our lives there."
- **Avoid the high fat foods** such as oleomargarine, uncooked dressings (mayonnaise, french dressing), heavy pastries, fish packed in oil, the hydrogenated shortenings, and cooked nuts. Use butter sparingly. Use fresh foods preferably. If these are not available, use frozen ones. If at all possible, do not use canned or boxed foods.
- **Eliminate milk and milk products from the diet.** I like the taste of milk, ice cream, and cheese, but I do not eat them! Neither should anyone else!
- **Prepare your food wisely.** Avoid fried food; instead bake, roast, broil, or boil meats. Eat as many raw vegetables as possible each day. When cooking vegetables, use as little water as possible, and start the vegetables in boiling water so that cooking time will be shorter. Do not overcook!
- **Work toward a good breakfast habit and noon-day meal.** Remember, the foods you eat during the day tend to be burned up during the day. When starchy foods are eaten at night, they are not used by the body for energy, but tend to be stored as fat!
- **Eat foods that can spoil**, but eat them before they spoil!

  By the way, how do you test to find out if bread is any good to eat? Take a slice or two of bread or any bread product. Put it on the top shelf of your kitchen cabinet. Allow it to stay there for 48 hours. Then take a look at it. If mold has developed on it, you can say "Oh, I have good bread!" Naturally, you want to eat it before it gets moldy. Mold only comes on something that is alive. If there is no mold on it, it's dead bread. It's been embalmed already.

Here is a story about shredded wheat; as told by Dr. Joe Nichols of Henderson, Texas. Dr. Nichols put an open box of shredded wheat in his garage and left it there for six months; no bugs or animals were interested in it. He then brought the open box into his office; it has been there for four years with no bugs; it is just as fresh as five years ago. In another experiment, he ground up the shredded wheat and fed it to a group of rats. He also ground up the box and fed it to another group of rats. In six months, the rats that ate the box were healthier.

- **Eat slowly**, masticate thoroughly, enjoy your food. Never overeat!
- **Eat in quiet.** Do not watch television or listen to talk shows on the radio. Quiet dinner music is fine.

Specific Food Recommendations

The following are specific recommendations in the various categories of foods indicated. **The left column lists approved, healthy foods, and the right column lists unhealthy foods to be avoided.** See Directions for Combining Foods on page 73 for suggestions on what foods may be eaten together to promote complete digestion.

Food and Diet

RECOMMENDED FOODS	FORBIDDEN FOODS
Beverages Chamomile tea, clear tea, mint tea, papaya tea, ginseng tea, misc. herbal teas, Sanka, Pero, Postum Some acceptable ones are Soyalac (a milk substitute made from soybean); Pero, Cafix, Postum (all coffee substitutes), Sun-Gal, Yerba Mate, Mate, and herb and root teas (peppermint, rose hips, etc.).	**Beverages** Alcohol, cocoa, soft drinks, drinks that contain stimulants and depressants. Coffee, decaffeinated coffee, black tea, or any other drink that contains caffeine or acid are diuretics, and they break down kidney function. They also eliminate potassium and the vitamin B complex. **Drink absolutely no milk!**
Bread Rye, soya, whole wheat or bran muffins, whole wheat, sprouted grain	**Bread** All other, white enriched, bleached
Cereals Untoasted buckwheat, corn meal, cracked wheat, millet, steel-cut oatmeal, rice, sesame, fine ground grits, rye, 100% all bran, Vigor Whole grain cereals are superior and should be eaten raw, if possible. However, these may be cooked.	**Cereals** All other refined and bleached flour Corn and wheat should be avoided. Do not eat, under any circumstances, boxed cereals from the grocery store. Avoid processed grain foods such as macaroni, noodles, white rice, and spaghetti.

Cheese	Cheese
None	All forbidden
Dessert	**Dessert**
Fresh ripe fruit, stewed fruit, gelatin (made from naturally sweetened and colored fruit or fruit juice)	All pastries, puddings, custards, junket, sauces, Jello (artificially sweetened and colored), ice cream
Fruit and gelatin salads are acceptable, but not when made with Jello. One should use unsweetened, uncolored, and unflavored gelatin and add fruit and fruit juices.	Eat absolutely no pastries, custards, puddings, candy, or ice cream!
Eggs	**Eggs**
Soft boiled or poached from chickens raised on the ground	In any form from caged chickens
Fats and Oils	**Fats and Oils**
Butter (unsalted), cold-pressed, unsalted oils such as olive, corn, sesame, sunflower, safflower	Oleomargarine
	Shortening, saturated fats and oils
Only a few of commonly available oils are acceptable for use. The best ones, listed in the order of their acceptability are sesame, flaxseed, sunflower, soy, cottonseed, olive, and corn.	**Avoid all fried foods; they contain dehydrogenated oils.**
	Mayonnaise and prepared, bottled dressings
The best healthy dressing is one made with cider vinegar and unsaturated oil. Honey may be added as a natural sweetener, and herbs may be used to flavor the mixture.	Canola oil
	(**Editor:** Dr. Ellis' recommendations were made before canola (rapeseed) oil became popular. Some cautions about ingestion of rapeseed oil are found at http://breathing.com/articles/canola-oil.htm, and http://www.diabetesincontrol.com/component/content/article/64-feature-writer-article/2570&Itemid=8.)
	Peanut oil (allergenic)

Food and Diet

Fish	Fish
Fresh, white-fleshed, salt-water top feeders	All fresh-water, salt-water bottom feeders
Vegetables	**Vegetables**
Raw, frozen, fresh or freshly cooked: artichokes, asparagus, carrots, cauliflower, celery, chives, corn, endive, green leeks, spinach, green peas, green pepper, lentils, lima beans, potatoes, radishes, tomatoes, wax beans, string beans, yams, egg plant, squash, mushrooms, beets, sprouts, mung beans, raw dandelion greens, beet greens, broccoli, Brussels sprouts, raw cabbage, cucumber (unpeeled), lettuce, washed sauerkraut, raw spinach (never cooked), parsley, rutabaga, Swiss chard, onions, turnips, and potatoes (used sparingly, not over once a week)

Any vegetables listed under salads

Vegetables may be eaten raw or cooked, but cooking should be done with as little water as possible as in wok cookery. Cooking in this sense could be best described as "wilting."

Use cayenne pepper and organic garlic, as well as onions. They do not cause digestive problems. | All canned

Spices and contents such as black and red peppers or hot peppers. They destroy stomach acidity. |

Fruit	Fruit
Fresh fruit or water-packed only and preferably between meals, including: apples, pears, apricots, cherries, currants, grapes, guava, mangos, melons, nectarines, papaya, peaches, plums, quince, tangerines, avocados, ripe pineapple, rhubarb, grapefruit and oranges (once a week if the system tolerates), lemons, currants, gooseberries, strawberries, cranberries, blueberries, loganberries, blackberries, raspberries. Fruit is best eaten singly and separately at least three hours after you've had protein. The following dried, unsulfured fruit can be stewed: apples, apricots, dates, figs, prunes, peaches, pears, plums, raisins, dates, apricots. Eaten only very ripe: bananas (use sparingly because they are highly alkalizing) Do not eat acidic and alkaline fruit together.	Canned fruit because they are preserved in sugar. The so-called dietetic fruit are just as bad with their chemical sugar substitute.

Food and Diet

Juices	Juices
Only fresh juices, consumed within minutes after being made for the best results. These may be selected from lists of permitted fruit and vegetables, including the following green leaves: chicory, endive, escarole, lettuce, Swiss chard, and watercress. Prune and cranberry juices (truly acidic, from malic acid) are better for us as we get older. Vegetable and unsweetened fruit juices are acceptable, but not when packed in metal or plastic. The preferred containers are glass.	All canned juices, and juices with artificial coloring and sweetening Tomato and tomato juice based drinks should be avoided, as should citrus juices.
Meat	**Meat**
Lean, grilled, broiled, roasted or baked beef, chicken and turkey (raised on the ground), lamb, and veal. Internal organs: only heart and extra fresh calf liver permitted. Meats should be prepared by broiling at 280° F. They should never be eaten well done; they should be eaten as rare as possible.	Bacon, ham, sausage, or pork, most of which are preserved with chemicals, especially nitrates or nitrites. They form the carcinogen classes of nitrosamines, a most potent cancer causer. Cold cuts, luncheon meats, canned meats and hot dogs; as they have the same preservatives, and most of them contain red dye. Smoked or barbecued meats. They are also cancer causers. Beef that has fat in the lining portion of the muscle. This means that the animal was raised on hormones and antibiotics. Do not eat chickens that are raised on wire — the cages.
Milk and Milk Products Butter	**Milk and Milk Products** None except butter

Nuts	Nuts
All types of fresh raw nuts (avoid long term storage to minimize fungus growth; only 10 daily) Seeds and nuts of all kinds (except peanuts) are acceptable, but they should be eaten fresh, never cooked, especially in oil, and in moderation, with no salt, no preservatives, and in moderation.	Roasted and salted Peanuts (allergenic)
Potatoes	**Potatoes**
Baked, boiled and mashed, potato salad, brown rice or corn as a substitute	French fries, shoestring, pan fried, white rice
Salads	**Salads**
The following raw vegetables, shredded or finely chopped, separated or mixed: carrots, cauliflower, celery, chicory, green pepper, lettuce, radishes, Swiss chard, watercress, onions, ripe tomatoes, turnips, Brussels sprouts, broccoli	Any salad with fatty or sweetened dressing
Seasoning	**Seasoning**
Chives, garlic, onion, cayenne pepper, parsley; herbs such as laurel, marjoram, sage, thyme, savory, cumin, oregano; salt substitutes such as Cosalt or other potassium salt	Black pepper, paprika, sodium salt
Soup	**Soup**
Vegetable, barley, brown rice, wild rice, millet	Canned and creamed soup, fat stock, consomme
Sweets	**Sweets**
Unpasteurized honey, unsulfured molasses, raw sugar, or dark brown sugar, carob	Candy, chocolate, white sugar

> Any variations in this diet should be done only with a doctor's permission.
>
> Avoid all toxic materials including alcohol and tobacco. Keep away from other people that smoke.

Meat

My favorite meal is nothing but a nice piece of meat and a nice raw vegetable salad, using apple cider vinegar (don't use any other kind of vinegar) with a good oil like sesame oil, sunflower oil, or a good olive oil. I like sesame because it has vitamin T in it to support blood platelets.

One of the big problems with protein in the diet is that so few people know how to cook proteins. We have been teaching what the Pennsylvania Restaurant Association taught us. These professionals did the research on how you should cook meat to get the most good out of it.

Correct Cooking Temperatures

Meat should be cooked at an internal temperature of 138° F. Use a meat thermometer for accuracy. It just takes a little longer. This temperature is in the range of minimum pasteurization temperatures, depending on the length of the cooling time.

Editor: Below is a helpful chart of cooking temperature and time combinations to ensure pasteurization of beef, lamb, and pork from Amazingribs.com. For data on other meats, visit the website.

Table 1: Meat Cooking Temperature vs. Cooking Time

Internal Temperature (°F)	Cooking Time
130	121 minutes
135	37 minutes
140	12 minutes
145	4 minutes
150	72 seconds
155	23 seconds
158	0 seconds

Most people today and most restaurants, cook meat at an external temperature of 350-400° F, which often carries the internal temperature of the meat too high, robbing it of vital, nutritious juices and making it tougher to digest. Meat juice is the plasma of the cell; it is not blood. When I started in this business many years ago, we didn't have the protein supplements like we can get today at the health food stores. The meat juice remains valuable.

One of the few times that I have ever agreed with the FDA comes from an article in the *Wall Street Journal* of August 1977; it says, "Blood rare beef pre-cooked to fade from the food counters. US to order that the meat be cooked to 145° F."

145° F is pretty close to 138° F, and to have the FDA finally admit this shows that we people in the health field really have something! 145° F does kill the Salmonella, or any other bacteria if it is cooked like that, and you get the temperature on the inside to 138° F and that's when you eat it.

Suggested Cooking Sequence

Here are some stepwise instructions that will help you learn how to cook beef, lamb, and pork properly.

- Depending on the thickness of the meat, select a cooking time that ensures the entire piece will be cooked to completion at the desired internal temperature. You must monitor the internal temperature of the meat with a meat thermometer.
- Rinse the meat and allow it to attain room temperature, but do not let it sit at room temperature very long; otherwise bacteria

will multiply, making your job more difficult. Do not salt the meat before cooking!

- Preheat the oven to the desired external temperature. Start with 250° F; put the meat in the oven.
- Allow the meat to warm up as long as necessary for the internal temperature to reach 138° F. To measure the temperature, insert a meat thermometer into the thickest portion of the meat and take a reading for no more than 15 seconds. (Instant-read thermometers are not oven safe and must not be left in the meat while it is cooking.)
- When the internal temperature reaches 138° F, start timing the cooking period. Adjust the external temperature as necessary to maintain the internal temperature.
- At the end of the recommended cooking time, take the meat out of the oven and heat the oven to broiling temperature.
- Put the meat back in the oven and let the broiler sear the surface, creating a crust that will hold in the juices. Let it cook for two to three minutes; the internal temp should remain at 138° F.
- When the crust is formed, pull the meat from the oven. Do not cut it immediately! Let it rest for at least 15 to 30 minutes to allow the juices to finish circulating and settle. The internal temperature of the meat will rise 3-5° F during this time.

Editor: Foodnetwork.com states, "Ground meat is riskier, because a contaminated meat surface is broken into small fragments and spread through the mass. The interior of a raw hamburger usually does contain bacteria, and is safest if cooked well done." Escherichia coli (E. coli) is killed at 155° F, but the USDA minimum safe internal temperature for ground beef is 160° F. Read more at: http://www.foodnetwork.com/recipes/articles/meat-and-poultry-temperature-guide.html?oc = linkback.

Microwave Cooking

What happens to meat in a microwave oven? The protein on the inside is devitalized. The U.S. government did a study of two groups of men for 90 days one group ate microwaved food and the other ate food cooked by conventional means. At the end of 60 days the men that ate the microwaved food were so tired and listless they got rid of the microwave ovens. There is also a radiation factor; read Linda Clark's *Are You Radioactive?* Food cooked in a microwave oven is devitaminized because it cooks at 2,000° F. The food is also demineralized, as indicated by the low values shown in a hair mineral analysis.

The microwave sets up free radicals, better known as peroxides. When eating microwave cooked food, you may just as well reach over and drink a bottle of hydrogen peroxide; it is exactly the same thing.

Pressure Cooking

Keep the heat as low as possible.

Barbecue Cooking

Although barbecued meat should be avoided, if one must eat some occasionally, ensure that the heat source is not directly under the food to be cooked. Meat drippings should not be burned and vaporized so that they come in contact with the meat.

Eggs

Eggs are one of the finest protein foods that you can eat. It is a complete protein, but you must know something about them. In the first place, they must be fertile, which means there must have been a rooster around for every 12 hens when those eggs were made, and when you put it in an incubator it could make another chick. They must come from chickens that are raised on the ground and not in cages (on wire). Wire makes it easy for the farmer because all of the droppings go down underneath and are easy to pick up. It's a little more difficult when they're on the ground. But when they are on the ground, they're picking up the gravel which goes into their craws, which is their digestive enzyme system. They pick up the bugs, worms, and all of these things that give them proper nourishment, to make a good egg.

The most important thing to remember is that under the shell of an egg is an enzyme called avidin. If you crack the shell of an egg, avidin destroys the biotin and the pantothenic acid, the two most important parts of the egg. It also neutralizes the lecithin, which is very high in eggs. Place it in boiling water for 30 seconds to deactivate the avidin and kill the bacteria under the shell. If you scramble or fry an egg or put it in an omelet and you're using grease, it's those oils and fats that become polysaturated; you destroy the lecithin and have an unbalanced egg that is harmful.

Food and Diet

Editor: In a study published by Durance, T. D. (1991). *Residual Avidin Activity in Cooked Egg White Assayed with Improved Sensitivity. Journal of Food Science.* 56 (3): 707-9. doi:10.1111/j.1365-2621.1991.tb05361.x. A new assay method found residual avidin activity in fried, poached, and boiled (2 minute) egg white to be 33%, 71%, and 40% of the activity in raw egg white. This suggested that cooking times were not sufficient to adequately heat all cold spot areas within the egg white. Complete inactivation of avidin's biotin binding capacity required boiling for over 4 minutes.

Dr. Emmanual Cheraskin at the University of Alabama took a group of dentists whose cholesterols ranged from 600 to well over 1,500 mg%. He wanted them less than two hundred, preferably under 175. On the scale he was using the low normal was 150. He put them on six soft boiled eggs every day. In 90 days, every one of their cholesterols were reduced to less than 200, and most of them were less than 175. You see, proteins burn up cholesterol. Now where does cholesterol come from? Cholesterol is manufactured through the colon and the liver from starches, sugar, and milk products. Less than 15% comes from foods that contain cholesterol, so don't be taken in by the advertising gimmicks they put on television and radio.

Again, make sure your eggs come from chickens raised on the ground not on wire; 95% are raised on wire. These chickens are loaded with a microorganism called by Dr. Virginia Livingston the Progenitor cryptocides (see Additional Reading on page 195); which are found in all people with cancer. To her, it is one of the basic causes of cancer. All people that I know with cancer cannot digest meat properly, so it putrefies and causes cell degeneration. They need HCl, trypsin, and chymotrypsin.

Fats

Unsaturated oils are preferred, and the best is sesame. The linoleic, oleic, and arachidonic acids are highest in sesame oil. The next best is safflower, followed by sunflower oil. In sesame oil is vitamin T; it builds blood platelets required for clotting. You can mix 1/2-1 cup of these oils with butter and keep the mixture in the refrigerator or freezer. At room temperature, It can turn rancid long before you can taste or smell it.

Editor: Dr. Ellis' recommendations were made before canola (rapeseed) oil became popular. Some cautions about ingestion of rapeseed oil are

found at http://breathing.com/articles/canola-oil.htm, and http://
www.diabetesincontrol.com/component/content/article/64-feature-
writer-article/2570&Itemid=8.

Vegetables

There are 65 green, yellow, and red vegetables. Take 10 or 12 of these, and
put them through a salad maker. If the particles are very small you won't
get into so much trouble because you won't have to chew 40-50 times. It is
very rare that I can get anybody to chew more than 5-10 times. It is a case
of attacking their food rather than chewing it properly. It is vital to do
enough chewing to get the saliva to mix with the food, because it activates
the production of hydrochloric acid in your stomach.

Parsley, by the way, is one of the great vegetables that we have, with
probably more vitamins and minerals than any other vegetables. Another, if
you want to get some potassium, is a raw potato. However, eating from the
nightshade family, of which the potato is a member, might increase pain for
a person who is arthritic. The part of the potato you want to eat is the skin
and the 1/4" under it. That is where the food value is located. The inside is
pure starch. If you go to a banquet, where you usually end up with a baked
potato and meat, take a spoon, and scoop out the inside of the potato and
throw that away. Eat the remainder, and it won't be so harmful to you.

Fruit - Good or Bad?

All fruits are good if they are tree-ripened. There are only four acid residue
fruit: prunes, plums, cranberries, and rhubarb. Rhubarb must be eaten raw
because it's high in oxalic acid. If cooked, it interferes with calcium
metabolism in the body. If it is sour there are insufficient minerals. Rhubarb
is sweet and delicious raw.

Acid fruit can be mixed with anything with the exception of alkaline fruit.
All other fruit, including tomatoes, leave an alkaline residue. Alkaline fruits
are best eaten singly, all by themselves at least three hours after or two
hours before eating protein. All fruit is to be eaten between meals and
before bedtime if very hungry.

My favorites are grapefruit, oranges, apples, and bananas. Two of those are
good, and two are not so good. Citrus is picked green and shipped to you;
that's what you buy. It took me six months of fighting with the Florida Citrus
Commission to make them agree that there wasn't any vitamin C in oranges.
You get vitamin C only from tree-ripened fruit.

The most important thing about bananas is that the skin is real thin. When we were in the Caribbean, I paid a kid fifty cents to go up a tree and get me a banana that was tree ripened. You wouldn't believe the difference in the flavor of that one banana compared to what you have in the stores. All bananas are picked green, then they are shipped to the destination, where they are put into a gas chamber to turn them yellow. Then we think that they are ripe. But, as long as those skins are thick, they are still green. Buy your bananas this week off the stand and eat them next week or the week afterwards. Let the enzymes in the skin work on the banana to ripen it. When they get a lot of black marks all over is when you eat them; then you can use the potassium effectively. Other sources of potassium are avocados and parsley.

Tomatoes - A Fruit to Avoid

Many authors call tomatoes the golden fruit with many vitamins. But I don't believe it. In Ireland, they grow the most beautiful, perfect tomatoes with plants 10 feet high with small tomatoes on them. We went from there to the Soviet Union and Switzerland, and in every country, they would serve you tomatoes and cucumbers for lunch and supper. I eat neither of them, but if you do, remember to eat cucumbers with the green covering on the outside, as that's where the enzyme factors are. If you peel it, you lose all of that and the cucumber is more harmful to you at that particular time. **A cancerous person should not eat tomatoes, it will neutralize the treatment and make the cancer worse.**

Cleaning Vegetables and Fruit

Today we are running into a lot of arsenical poisonings because of the sprays being put upon your vegetables. So when I talk about the sprays put on vegetables, let me teach you how to make sure they are fit for you to eat. All of your fruit and vegetables today, practically all of them, have some kinds of pesticides or weedicides, or some other type of spray on them. To remove them, follow these instructions.

- Use plain, unscented household bleach; one tablespoon to a gallon of distilled water.

Editor: Bleach is very caustic; protect your eyes and wash it off of your skin immediately. Watch out for the safety of anyone around you, mop up spills, and do not leave the container open or exposed to children. Do not use spashless bleach; it foams extensively.

- Soak your fruit or vegetables for 15-20 minutes. This will remove most of these pesticides, weedicides, and sprays from the outside.
- Take them out, dry them, and put them into distilled water for another fifteen minutes. This will remove the rest of the residue.

Make the bleach water new each time and throw it out after you finish with it. It works out a whole lot better that way.

A Sample Menu for the Day

Our research has proven that our finest health menus consist of 50% or more protein in our diet; 20% or less of fats, mostly from unsaturated oils, and 30% carbohydrates, mostly from green, red, and yellow vegetables and not heavy starches.

To maintain best health, the largest meal of the day should be breakfast, as that is the energy you work on all of the rest of the day. The second largest meal should be lunch, and the evening meal should be small. This is so that the gastrointestinal tract can have some rest while you sleep. Eat no snacks in the evening. If this order is reversed, I can predict weight gain. Another point to be made is to eat natural foods whenever possible.

Table 2 is a sample menu showing you that it is possible to serve a day's meals that are high in protein, low in fat, and that supply nutrients that add up to better health. There are, of course, many variations; substitutions may be made from the foods listed under Specific Food Recommendations on page 57. There is, however, no substitute for the gelatin.

Table 2:   Sample Menu for the Day

Meal or Snack	Components
Breakfast	Select either of the following: • Prune or cranberry juice upon arising, one or two eggs (soft boiled or soft poached), one or two slices of whole grain bread, and a beverage from those listed in the previous chart. (Bread and its products are not usually recommended in combination with a protein food. However, soft boiled or soft poached eggs are digestible when eaten with a moderate portion of whole grain bread, preferably toasted. The same statement cannot be made for meat proteins or eggs that are cooked to a hard consistency.) • Cooked whole grain cereal, honey if desired, cranberry or prune juice, choice of a beverage from those listed in the previous chart.
Mid-Morning	Fruit juice or cold water with one package of gelatin added.
Lunch (sometimes called Dinner)	Broiled ground beef patties (cooked rare to medium rare), raw vegetable salad with dressing, choice of beverage.
Mid Afternoon	Fresh fruit
Dinner (sometimes called Supper)	Vegetable soup with Rye Crisp, choice of meat (prepared as above), vegetables, cole slaw, or salad with dressing; choice of beverage.
Bedtime	For a relaxing sleep, drink cranberry juice, warm bouillon, or cold water to which has been added a package of gelatin.

When I'm on the road I eat mostly soft boiled eggs. There's another thing that you can do with an egg. If you take a raw egg from the icebox, warm it up a little bit under the faucet with warm water then put it into boiling water for 30 seconds to destroy the avidin enzyme. Crack the shell and combine them with cranberry juice in a blender (8 ounces). That is a meal. The acidity of the cranberry juice picks all of the acidity out of the egg so that you would not know it is raw. Cranberry juice, being acid (malic acid that does not break down in the body), helps to digest the protein. You can also add one tablespoon of gelatin. It's an excellent meal. You can also use prune juice, which also contains malic acid. Many times, when I am sitting at home writing my 30-35 letters a day, I don't have much time to take off for lunch, so I'll make this delicious drink, and I'm good for five hours.

When I'm at home I like my organically grown rye, millet, and steel-cut oatmeal. Usually what I do is take a tablespoon of buckwheat, a cup of rye, and a cup of millet. They are the highest in minerals and protein of all cereals. I put it in a double boiler with two cups of distilled water, because no city water that I know of is fit to drink anywhere. While it's cooking, I put it on a low temperature and shave, shower, and dress. That gives me about 25 minutes to finish; I come back to the kitchen and put cranberry juice in the mixture. It's very delicious and lasts me about five to six hours.

You could probably use raw bran, barley, or brown or wild rice as a cereal. Then you don't eat anything else that's all you need at that particular time. Lunches and suppers remain somewhat the same. Of course we have some kind of meat. I would advise at least seven to 21 meals from salt water fish.

Directions for Combining Foods

Proper combining of foods optimizes the digestive processes. **It is possible to eat a variety of foods that interfere with the digestion of certain others. Likewise, it is possible to eat foods that enhance the digestion or, at least, do not interfere with the digestion of the others.** Properly and completely digested carbohydrates yield monosaccharides; improperly and incompletely digested carbohydrates yield the poisonous substances acetic acid and alcohol (fermentation). Completely digested proteins yield amino acids, whereas incompletely digested proteins yield ptomaines and leucomaines (putrefaction), both poisonous substances.

Allergies are a manifestation of improperly digested proteins that enter the bloodstream before they are broken into a sufficiently small fragment; such reactions can be prevented by effecting the eating habits that promote the most efficient digestion all along the alimentary canal. Some suggestions are as follows.

- **Select your proteins wisely.**
  Muscle meat is difficult to digest, even when combined properly with other foods. The best and most digestible source of protein is the egg, and it should be soft boiled or soft poached; never fried, scrambled, or hard boiled.

- **Do not mix proteins with starches (carbohydrates).**
  As proteins move into the stomach, pepsin is secreted, and this triggers the release of hydrochloric acid. Protein digestion requires this acidic environment. However, as the medium becomes more and more acidic, carbohydrate digestion becomes curtailed. Furthermore, the presence of the carbohydrate neutralizes the acid; i.e., the medium that is favorable to the digestion of one is unfavorable to the digestion of the other. Meat and potatoes is, therefore, a poor combination, as is meat and alkaline fruit, starches, and sugars.
- **Do not mix acid (alkaline-forming) fruit with proteins.**
  Alkaline fruit include tomatoes and all fruit except prunes, plums, cranberries, and rhubarb. These should be eaten singly and at least three hours after ingestion of proteins. Acid (acid-forming) fruit, such as prunes, plums, cranberries, and rhubarb, can aid digestion and can be used in the same meal as protein foods. (Rhubarb contains oxalic acid and, on that basis, should be avoided.)
- **Do not mix acid (alkaline-forming) fruit with starches.**
  Citrus fruit or vinegar will inhibit the action of ptyalin, a starch digesting enzyme that originates in salivary secretions. It will not act in even a mildly acidic medium. Proper chewing assures mixing of foods with ptyalin, but the enzyme can become inactivated upon contact with the ingested acids and not be able to work before gastric hydrochloric acid is secreted.
- **Do not mix sugars with starches.**
  Sugars, sweet fruit, and honey ferment if delayed in the stomach. Such a delay can occur if the sweets in the mouth inhibit the formation of ptyalin. This enzyme is necessary for the preparatory stages of starch digestion to trigger the movement on to the intestine where proper digestion of starches takes place. Do not drink sweetened drinks and eat breads at the same time.
- **Eat melons by themselves.**
  Melons are so simple to digest, they move directly to the intestine without inducing the formation of enzymes and hydrochloric acid. If other foods hold the melon in the stomach, it can ferment. It is acceptable to eat berries with melons.
- **Do not drink milk.**

Man is the only creature that drinks milk beyond the age of weaning. Milk causes mucous in the colon, allergies, and malabsorption of nutrients, and neutralizes the hydrochloric acid in the stomach. Milk should not, consequently, not be taken with any protein. The lesson is don't touch!

Food Combining Charts

The following two charts are for use in choosing foods for combination with each other in the same meal. Those boxes that are connected by lines may be combined. Do not combine foods if their boxes are not connected. For example, whenever you eat protein, meat, fish, fowl, eggs, gelatin, nuts, seeds, or cereal, do not eat bread, potatoes, lima beans, corn, or rice at the same time.

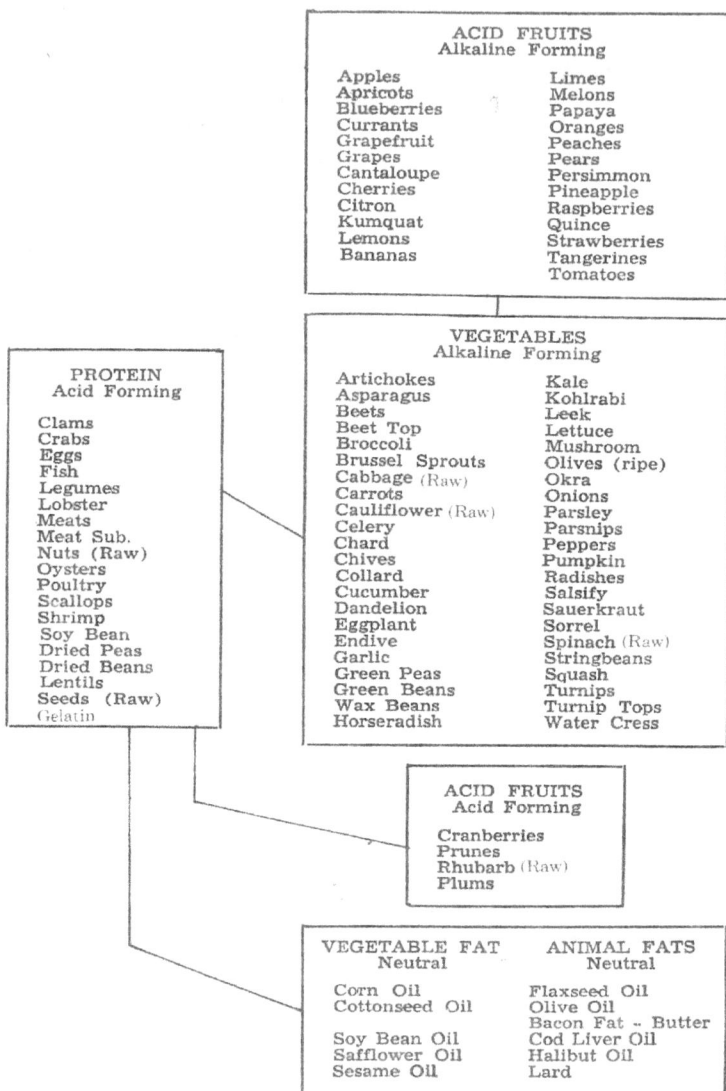

Figure 1: Combining proteins with other foods

STARCHES
Acid Forming
Barley
Beans (Kidney)
Beans (Lima)
Breads
Buckwheat
Cakes
Cereals
Chestnuts
Cookies
Corn
Crackers
Doughnuts
Flours
Lentils
Muffins
Peas (dried)
Pies
Potatoes (Irish)
Potatoes (Sweet)
Rolls
Rice (Brown)

VEGETABLES
Alkaline Forming

Artichokes	Kale
Asparagus	Kohlrabi
Beets	Leek
Beet Top	Lettuce
Broccoli	Mushroom
Brussel Sprouts	Olives (ripe)
Cabbage (Raw)	Okra
Carrots	Onions
Cauliflower (Raw)	Parsley
Celery	Parsnips
Chard	Peppers
Chives	Pumpkin
Collard	Radishes
Cucumber	Salsify
Dandelion	Sauerkraut
Eggplant	Sorrel
Endive	Spinach (Raw)
Garlic	Stringbeans
Green Peas	Squash
Green Beans	Turnips
Wax Beans	Turnip Tops
Horseradish	Water Cress

SUGAR
Acid Forming

Brown Sugar
Candy
Honey
Maple Syrup
Maple Sugar
Raw Sugar
White Sugar

SWEET FRUITS
Alkaline Forming

Dates
Dried Currants
Figs
Raisins

VEGETABLE FAT Neutral	ANIMAL FATS Neutral
Corn Oil	Sesame Oil
Cottonseed Oil	Flaxseed Oil
	Olive Oil
Soy Bean Oil	Bacon Fat - Butter
Safflower Oil	Cod Liver Oil
Sesame Oil	Halibut Oil
Safflower Oil	Lard - Egg Yolk

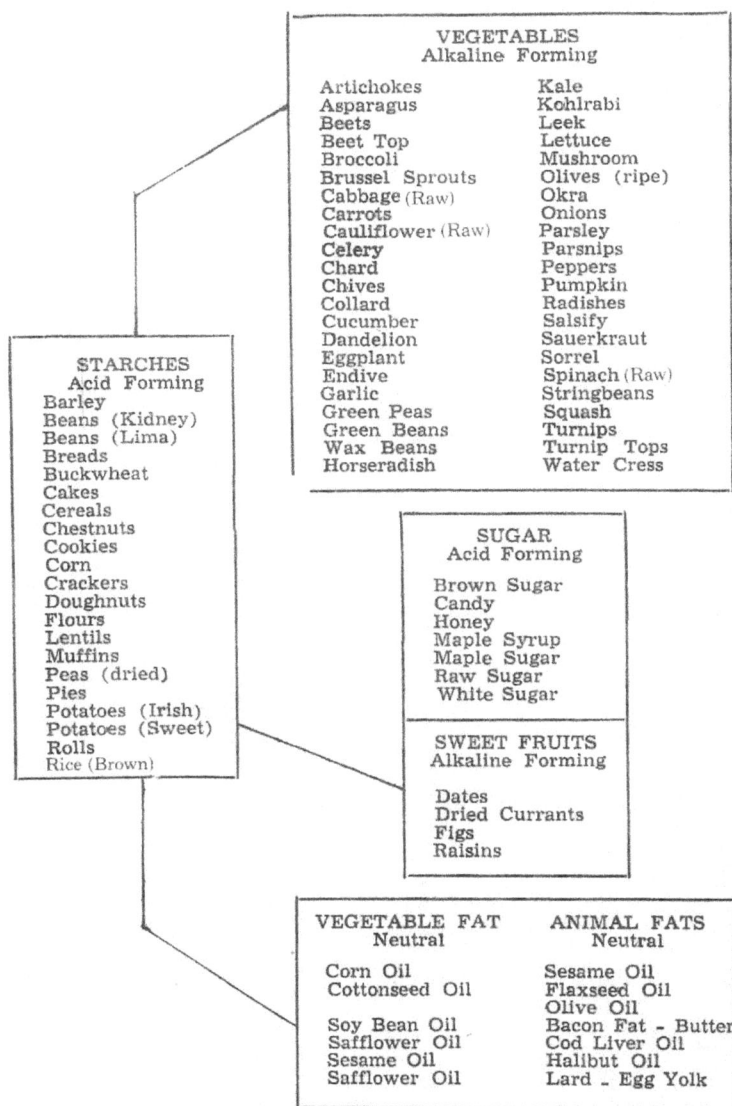

Figure 2: Combining starches with other foods

Food and Diet

4 The Water We Drink

I have checked cities in 40 states altogether, and I don't know of a city water supply that's fit for anybody to drink from. Even the Environmental Protection Agency (EPA) has shown that the city water of 89 of the largest cities in the United States has the potential to cause cancer.

What is contaminating the water supplies? Pollution from the air, nitrates and nitrites that farmers put on crops, and pesticides and herbicides that are being used. This amounts to chemical warfare; when the rain comes down where does it pour? Into our lakes and rivers; that's where we are taking the water for drinking. We're going to have to recycle our urine, feces, and everything else to get our water supply, if we don't look out. Because that's where we're going; it's up to each one of us to develop healthy priorities within ourselves and fight to remain healthy.

Making the Headlines

The headline in an article that I saw in a Pittsburgh newspaper says, *Tap water is inferior, the United States reports*. The information in this article was provided by the Department of Health, Education, and Welfare. To the side of the article, it states, "It was not unusual to find undesirable bacteria, arsenic, lead, barium, cadmium and other chemical delicacies in the tap water samples." Believe you me, when you start doing some checking on water, you will find how true it is, because we're doing it all of the time.

There are all kinds of unwanted contaminants in drinking water. For instance, the chemical element cadmium competes with and displaces zinc in the human metabolic processes. Excess cadmium provokes high blood pressure. One place where you pick up cadmium is in your drinking water, the other place is from smoking cigarettes. **Almost everyone in the United States is being poisoned by some type of metal pollutant.**

This is the work of Dr. Henry A. Schroeder, who probably knew more about minerals and their activity within the human body than anyone else that I know of. One of the most important additives to water that we are watching today is chlorine; a cancer link is claimed. When pesticides, weedicides, nitrates, and nitrites are present in the water supply, the added chlorine combines with many of these chemicals and sets up a chloroform type of chemical that is a carcinogen.

Never use softened water for drinking purposes; the salt or the chemicals that are put in can be most harmful to the human body. The salt gets in there and throws the balance of sodium and potassium right out of line. It gets you into all kinds of problems, so we tell you very definitely to stay away from it.

Editor: For current information on contaminants in water supplies, see http://water.usgs.gov/nawqa/studies/domestic_wells/.

The Politics of Water

I had a patient that used to come in with vague aches and pains as if he was getting a slight cold, runny nose. I'd get them cleared up and he would be good for maybe two, three, four weeks. Then, he would be back in the office for the same thing all over again. This went on for about six months and I said, "I'd like you to bring me a sample of your water." Now his family lived out in the country, on the side of a hill. He said, "What's the matter? Our water tastes real good. It looks clear you know, nice sandy type of loam out there; everything's fine." I said, "I still want that sample; I'm going to have it analyzed." Which I did.

The analysis came back stating that his water was unfit for human consumption. So we decided to do a little investigating. We found out that six months earlier, on the opposite side of this hill, a new house had been put in, and the septic tank apparently wasn't installed properly, because the overflow started early. It went into the underground water supply that was going through the hill and came up into the opposite side of the hill, where my patient lived.

Of course, from then on we knew what the answer was; they would have to boil it. The only thing that was wrong was the bacteria. So if they use this water for humans or animals, they would have to boil this water, or drill a new well somewhere else, to get away from those bacteria.

Disaster in the Mouth

If true preventive dentistry were more widely practiced, the American mouth would not be the disaster area that it is. More than 25 million people put their choppers in a glass every night. 95% have cavities — more than one billion cavities and 75% have gum disease. Dental problems are proliferating faster than the nation's dentists can cope with them.

When you get this kind of report, you realize that fluoridated toothpastes aren't stopping cavities, and they don't. They actually do more damage to the gums. If you want to do the best thing, never scrub your teeth. You should never put a toothbrush on them. What you should scrub, is the gums. Get that circulation into that gum, then you won't have that problem with cavitation. Also stay off of sugar.

Rats given fluoride in their drinking water at levels as low as in some cities water systems developed abnormalities that led to miscarriages, still births, and birth defects. One other little thing, fluoride poisoning as a result of ingesting fluoride salts is a serious environmental hazard for both children and adults. Inhalation results in inflammatory changes in the lungs that can progress to pulmonary emphysema. In systemic absorption, the ion binds to circulating calcium causing severe hypocalcemia, tetany, and cardiac arrhythmias. Laundry powders may be one of the main sources of fluoride.

Fluoridation of Public Water Supply

Probably the big one that we talk about most is the work of Dr. Dean Burk, the former head of the cancer division, of the National Cancer Institute in Washington. I don't know much about the use of fluoridation in Canada, but I do know that some of the research done in Toronto and Montreal has shown that if fluoridated water is used for a person on a kidney machine, the patient is always dead within 24 hours. The medical school in Toronto took a look at children between the ages of four and sixteen who were using fluoride toothpaste to stop cavitations in teeth. They found out that these children swallowed between 20% and 26% of the toothpaste.

Dr. Ali H. Mohammed at the University of Missouri, Kansas City, said, "Cities began adding fluoride to their water supply 20-25 years ago and now some 95 million are drinking artificially fluoridated water." Let's do a little interesting mathematics. Early on, the United States Government, mandated one part per million (ppm) of fluoride in drinking water. They have now reduced it to 0.75 ppm. But for illustration, let's use one ppm; it's easier mathematics. If children swallow a portion of the toothpaste that most everybody is using these days, all users are going to consume additional fluoride. All canned vegetables are packed in fluoridated water, at least they are in the states. Add this to the fluoride that is coming from air pollution, and it is an impossibility for your body to stay at even one ppm; therefore the actual level becomes poisonous. **One thing of great interest to me is that fluoridated water destroys the production of hydrochloric acid in your stomach, an absolute necessity for digesting food, and it antagonizes iodine, needed by a variety of tissues.**

The Fluoride Movement

The fluoride movement was started by a dentist in Deaf Smith County, Texas. He had found that their water was pretty high in calcium fluoride. He wasn't a biochemist, so he didn't realize that calcium fluoride is the natural or organic form. He didn't see that many cavities around there, so he gave credit to it. **The corporations picked this up, because the end product of aluminum manufacturing is the inorganic form of fluoride, sodium silica fluoride.** The only good that it was ever used for was rat poisoning and for etching glass. They had stock piles of it all over the place and didn't know what to do with it to get rid of it. So they hooked onto the idea of this dentist. **They let everybody believe that the inorganic fluorides were the same as the organic fluorides, which is 100% wrong!** Today you're seeing stannous fluorides; these are all in the inorganic form, and that's why they are so harmful to the human body. They make your bones brittle.

Distilled Water

We tell you today, to drink distilled water. Now we hear a lot of people say, "Drinking distilled water demineralizes you." Well, this is not true, there is no research that proves this. The one thing that it doesn't do for you is give you the necessary minerals. As a result of not giving them to you, you can have a depletion occur in the body. That's why we tell you to have a hair analysis to tell you what your minerals are doing in your body. Then, you supplement to your mineral deficiencies. With respect to distillers, I think one of the better ones today, is this New World distiller. It takes little space, and you can hook it right up to your water supply and let it run on a constant basis.

Editor: The New World Distiller Corporation of Gravette, Arkansas is no longer in business. It is suggested that the reader review the selection of

distillers on the internet, beginning with http://
www.purewaterinc.com/Shop-Water-Distillers.

The Water We Drink

5   Milk and Milk Products

I believe that milk and milk products are the number one cause of disease! I have found it to be the leading cause of colds, sinus conditions, asthma, bronchitis, and mucous colitis. No moo for you!

Milk is a product made by a human or animal mother to supply adequate food for her offspring. This milk is intended to be the baby's food until its own digestive enzymes begin to be produced in sufficient quantity to digest solid food. When the transfer is appropriate, the mother's breasts dry up and return to their normal size. The cow does the same thing for its calf as a mother does for her baby — if left alone within her natural habitat.

The first recorded incidence of an infant being given cow's milk was in 1793. Since then, many articles have been written, stating that milk is the perfect food for man, supplying all or most of his daily needs. Included among these publications are magazines such as *Life* and *Time*, as well as nutritional periodicals and even literature published by the Department of Agriculture.

I've performed more than 25,000 blood tests for my patients. These tests show conclusively, in my opinion, that adults who use milk products do not absorb nutrients as well as adults who don't. Of course, poor absorption, in turn, means chronic fatigue.

Jefferson Medical College in Philadelphia, in a course on heart attacks and strokes, taught that they have found that milk and milk products to be the greatest single cause of heart attacks in humans. Because of its mucous formation it can be one of the main causes of crib deaths. Milk forms mucous, giving the baby a hard time breathing: they twist and turn getting the bedclothes all over themselves, but they actually suffocate from the mucous in the bronchial tubes. It is published that 30,000 deaths a year are due to milk and milk products.

Doctor to Patient

Dr. Lynn Ferguson of the Ferguson-Droste-Ferguson Rectal Hospital in Grand Rapids, Michigan, stated before a group at the American Medical Association meeting in 1961, that they would have to close the doors of their 200 bed hospital within a year if all people stopped using milk and milk products. If you take it on a daily basis, you have your body so poisoned that you don't realize what these symptoms are that are hitting you. But if you stay away from it for 90 days and then try it, you will find out how fast it really hits you.

Milk is the greatest cause of human disease that I know of. I have challenged every milk industry in the world to prove on a scientific basis that cow's milk or goat's milk can be used on human beings without harm. So far, not one of them have accepted my challenge.

Editor: For a recent review on the role of dairy products in the human diet, see *Dairy: Milking It for All It's Worth* by Dr. Loren Cordain, author of *The Paleo Diet* at http://thepaleodiet.com/dairy-milking-worth/. This article reviews the history of how milk became part of the human diet in conjunction with the domestication of animals 10,000 years ago. A short quote from this article reads as follows. "...we are the only species on the planet to consume another animal's milk throughout our adult lives. Humans don't have a nutritional requirement for the milk of another species, nor do any other mammals. An increasing body of scientific evidence supports the evolutionary caution that this dietary practice is not necessarily harmless."

Human vs. Cow's Milk

A calf has four stomachs; a human being, one. We humans simply do not possess the digestive enzymes found in the calf's third and fourth stomachs that allow him to digest milk. So, even if the milk is raw, we cannot digest it properly. Homogenized milk takes three or more hours to be digested and leave the stomach; a human mother's milk leaves the infant's stomach in less than 45 minutes.

The human baby develops his brain first, while the animal develops his bone structure first; therefore, milk for a human, and that for an animal naturally should be different. The calf develops his bone structure first and doubles his weight in the first 30 days. Approximately 90 pounds at birth, it will weigh 1,000 pounds at the end of its weaning period. Growing calves need more protein to enable them to grow quickly in size. Human infants, on the other hand, need less protein and more fat as their energies are expended primarily in the development of the brain, spinal cord, and nerves. In humans, the brain develops rapidly during the first year of life, growing faster than the body and tripling in size by the age of one.

Protein Content

The proteins in milk can be divided into two categories: casein and whey. 100 gm of whole cow's milk (3.3 gm) has more than double the protein of human milk (1.3 gm), and most of this protein is the soluble phosphoprotein, caseinogen. Cow's milk has a ratio of casein to whey proteins of 80:20, while human milk contains these in a ratio of 40:60, respectively. Problematically, in the stomach of human babies, caseinogen is converted by the enzyme rennin (before pepsin formation) to the insoluble casein, a form more difficult for babies to digest.

Probably 50% or more of the protein in cow's milk is wasted. The sole purpose for rennin is milk digestion. As other digestive enzymes and hydrochloric acid appear, rennin disappears. Rennin leaves the human stomach by two years of age, at which time all milk and milk products should be stopped. The protein in human milk is lactalbumin which is soluble and easily digested. It is utilized by the baby easily, with virtually 100% efficiency. A baby raised on mother's milk will have more body flexibility and adaptability.

Fat Content

The total amount of fat in cow's milk is almost equal to that of human milk, but they differ in the type and proportions. Cow's milk contains more saturated fat while human milk contains more unsaturated fat, as shown in Table 3.

Table 3:   Comparison of Fat Content, Bovine vs. Human Milk

Proportion of Types of Fat in Milk British Food Standards Agency (FSA)	
100 gm of Cow's Milk	**100 gm of Human Milk**
2.5 gm saturated	1.8 gm saturated
1.0 gm monounsaturated	1.6 gm monounsaturated
0.1 gm polyunsaturated	0.5 gm polyunsaturated

The higher level of unsaturated fatty acids in human milk reflects the important role of these fats in brain development. The brain is largely composed of fat, and early brain development and function in humans requires a sufficient supply of polyunsaturated essential fatty acids. The omega-6 fatty acid, arachidonic acid (AA), and the omega-3 fatty acid, docosahexaenoic acid (DHA) are both essential for brain development and functioning. Both are generously supplied in human milk but not in cow's milk.

Other Nutrients

Although human milk contains less calcium than cow's milk, the calcium in human milk is better absorbed into the body than the calcium in cow's milk, again illustrating why human milk is the best source of nutrition during the first year of life. The best source of calcium depends on what you need. If you are going to build the immune system, the best source is calcium lactate. If you want to build the bones, the best source is raw veal bone.

The high protein, sodium, potassium, phosphorus, and chloride content of cow's milk present what is called a high renal solute load; this means that the unabsorbed solutes from the diet must be excreted via the kidneys. This can place a strain on immature kidneys forcing them to draw water from the body, thus increasing the risk of dehydration. Furthermore, cow's milk is low in vitamin C and vitamin D (Department of Health, 1994), and contains less vitamin A than human milk.

Importance of Breast Feeding

Mother's milk transfers immunity to the baby and implants enough intestinal bacteria to be the basis for a lifetime supply needed for resistance to infectious diseases. The most important milk, cow or human, is that milk produced in the first 10 hours after birth. The reasons it is important are threefold:

- Acidophilus bacilli are present for starting the normal intestinal flora for the intestinal tract. They are there only for the first 10 hours.

- An enzyme is present that activates the stomach and the intestinal tract to digest food. It starts all of the digestibility system of the cells. When we have separated calves from their mothers, milked the mothers, and then fed the milk out of the pan to the calves, those calves never develop like the ones that suckle off their mothers' nipples. The reason for it is that the enzyme in the nipple is there to help digest the milk. Air destroys that enzyme.

- A reflex mechanism that takes place during suckling makes the uterus contract, and thus stops the bleeding from the placental attachment area.

Humans are the only ones who do not know how to get from the birth canal to the breast of its mother. As soon as animals are born, they start wiggling and know exactly how to get to the nipples of their mothers. As soon as they get there, they start sucking. This applies to dogs, cats, calves, pigs, or anything else. Of course, that's the way that you are going to stop the mother from bleeding to death. You girls don't have to have that shot in the tail or pituitary extract to stop you from bleeding. All you have to do is put that baby on that breast, but it should be there within a matter of minutes. As soon as that cord stops pulsating, put a clamp on it, cut it, clean the face, and put the baby right up on the breast.

Children should be breast-fed as long as the mother can stand the teeth of the infant. They should get vegetables, etc., only after nine months to one year of age. The digestive enzyme ptyalin does not develop until six or seven months of age. **Some babies are being fed adult food in the first week; the food is not digested in the stomach, but its presence takes away the hunger feeling. They can get some colic and other problems, and this, in our opinion, is a major cause of disease in later life.**

Our research also shows that breast-fed babies do not run out of hydrochloric acid until they are near 50 years of age. Bottle-fed babies are running out in their late teens and twenties, and most are complete achlorhydrics by the time they reach 40 years of age. We know of one child four years of age that has no hydrochloric acid. When I did the analysis on this, I said to the doctor that this was a bottle-fed baby.

It was the first time that the doctor had heard me say that, so he wrote back, "How did you know?" It's very simple when you know this. Seventeen European researchers in 1972 published that the amino acid leucine in milk and milk products stimulated the beta cells of the Islets of Langerhans, causing an increase in insulin production. Thus, there is a basic cause for hypoglyemia. Continued use over a period of time breaks down the beta cells, causing diabetes.

Allergy to Milk

Today, in the United States, 28% of the food consumed is dairy. Up to 50% of whites, 75% of blacks, and 100% of orientals do not have the lactase enzyme in their bodies to handle lactose, the sugar that is in milk. Lactase is produced by the lining of the small intestine and in the majority of humans, this lactase production stops when weaning takes place in infancy. Only in Europe and America does this lactase production continue after weaning. When lactase production does stop, drinking of milk causes flatulence, bloating, and diarrhea. That is why milk is, in every book that I have looked at, number one on the allergy list. The other ones in the top five are chocolate, wheat, corn, and beef. Naturally, lactose-intolerant whites, blacks, and orientals should not touch milk in any form!

Milk is found to be loaded today with the same colon bacillus as found in the bowel. It lines all mucous membranes with excessive mucous, thus making absorption most difficult. Milk stimulates mucous membranes, so basically it is the main cause of colds, sinusitis, asthma, bronchitis, and mucous colitis. Most all degenerative diseases can be found to be more severe in those using milk or milk products. In most cheeses, also in chocolate, is an enzyme called phenylethylamine, and it is one of the main factors in producing migraine headaches.

Anything involving the lungs — sinus trouble, asthma, bronchitis — these are the things that are really basically allergies. Every allergy book you look at puts milk and milk products as number one on the list. **The only one thing that we want you to use is butter, because it does not have the enzymes or the hormones.**

I was brought before the Dairy Council in Michigan; their vice-president was my patient and was quite quiet, even though he was usually quite vociferous. It was getting to be time to vote on the question of suing me for the statements I was making, because I talk to many clubs, such as Rotary, Kiwanas, Exchange Club, and others.

One of the other members of the council suddenly realized and asked him why he hadn't said anything. He answered, "I just wanted to see how far you are going to go before you hang yourselves. I have had asthma for many years and I heard that this doctor treated differently than others and I have spent thousands of dollars trying to get rid of my asthma. I went to Dr. Ellis, who knew that I owned a dairy and was on the Dairy Council; he challenged me to go off milk products for 90 days and then go back and try one teaspoon of milk or ice cream or cheese. I accepted his challenge and, when I did try the teaspoon of milk, my asthma hit me in a matter of seconds. Then I had to go home and clean myself out again so I could get rid of it. This man knows more about milk than anyone on this Council. If you really want to make him and ruin the milk industry, you go ahead and sue him." They did not.

Pasteurization

Milk was supposedly pasteurized to destroy bacteria; however, for years, the law stated that raw milk could be sold with a bacterial count up to 10,000 bacteria per ml, but grade A pasteurized milk could be sold with a bacterial count up to 100,000 bacteria per ml, and grade B, 200,000. **Pasteurization is not done to destroy bacteria, it is done to destroy the phosphatase enzyme that helps to turn milk sour.** That is why today, with the destruction of the phosphatase enzyme, milk does not turn sour and therefore It does not need refrigeration.

Watch in the middle of the summer when your milk man goes down the street, you won't find any refrigeration on his truck, because he knows darn well that it won't turn sour. In fact, it won't even spoil with the new method. **Also, with the destruction of the phosphatase enzyme was the loss of our ability to assimilate calcium.** In pasteurization, lecithin is lost by the splitting of phosphorus salts. The casein alters its reaction and forms very hard curds. Some, like curds in skim milk take more than five hours to leave the stomach. The sugar of milk becomes caramelized, the citric acid is destroyed, the lime salts become insoluble, and the oxygen content is decreased.

Another of the major purposes of pasteurization of milk is to stabilize flavor. In the process, lysine becomes unavailable due to its incomplete enzymatic digestion and/or actual destruction in some cases. Milk for evaporation purposes is usually grade B, with a permitted bacteria count many times that of grade A milk. Pasteurization kills these bacteria, but it does not remove their dead bodies.

What has science shown? Two universities have found that good, strong calves, at about their second or third month, when taken off breast feeding and fed on their own mother's milk that had been pasteurized beforehand, died of heart attacks within eight months.

Some researchers have questioned the possible effects of pasteurization. Does it affect susceptible individuals, especially children, and cause diarrhea, nausea, or vomiting? Another serious question — since wheat and other grains are usually low in lysine and suffer biological change when heated, milk that is heated will not combine to provide a complete protein, as would otherwise result with unheated milk. When pasteurized or homogenized milk is used, this can pose a serious nutritional problem for millions of children.

Other Dairy Products

Ice cream is nothing more than a chemical concoction. It has a small amount of skim milk powder, and 34 chemicals including artificial colors and flavors that have been on the cancer causative list for at least 30 years. Recently the International Association of Cancer Victims and Friends published a list of all of these chemicals and what they do in the body. If you ever read that list you would never put another bit of ice cream in your mouth, believe me. It took the FDA eight years to get red dye #2 out of food, but now some companies have simply mixed it with another to make a new dye that is more poisonous, and still on the market. They are willing to put a chemical on the market and wait until the FDA tells them to stop. No drug should be put on the market until its manufacturer has researched to establish its safety.

Buttermilk today is made from skim milk with streptococcus lactic acid bacteria added. It is then incubated at a carefully controlled temperature until the right acidity is reached. Then, they add yellow butter flecks to some for visual effect. Cottage cheese, in the factory that I visited, is not the old-fashioned Smearcase as we old-timers knew it. Today they add bacteria to skim milk to make it curd. The curds are pulled off and washed with hippuric acid to destroy the bacteria. I don't know how many of you city folks have been around horses after they urinated, but that nice strong odor that you get out of that urine is hippuric acid; I just want to keep you up to date on all of these things! Then they add 13 chemicals, one of which is a drying agent very similar to plaster of paris, and what remains is sold to you as cottage cheese.

Yoghurt is in the same category. The milk that you get in yoghurt does more harm than the good that you get from the acidophilus bacilli. It's much simpler today to take freeze-dried acidophilus bacilli in a little tablet containing anywhere from six million to 100 million bacteria. You get the beneficial bacteria without milk allergens.

You see, to me anything that is 51% harmful and 49% good you had better stay away from, because it's going to add up and get you. And that's why I quit yoghurt and kefir both. One of my good friends Is the public relations man for a dairy company. He and I fight on this — lots of times on programs — he gets up and tells all of the virtues and good things about milk, and I get up and tell what I'm telling you about milk. So we really confuse the audience. I have found that it takes four days to get over the ill effects of one teaspoon full of any milk product, except butter, so I say to you, "Stay off all milk products for 90 days. Then just try one teaspoonful of milk, or ice cream, or a piece of cheese and watch how fast, within seconds, it clogs up your throat and nose with mucous and gives you a harder time breathing." It really does a job.

Butter is OK

Butter does not contain the enzymes and hormones found in other milk products. Never use axle grease (better known as margarine) anytime. It is too hard to digest. The leucine that stimulates insulin production in the B-cells of the Islets of Langerhans Is not found in butter, but only in milk. **Below is a direct quotation from *Margarine vs. Butter*, published in the *Lancet*, April 6, 1974.**

"The trend throughout the world today is to incorporate an ever-increasing amount of the polyunsaturated fats into human diets. And there is considerable evidence that this practice is not exactly contributing to a glorious old age. Quite the contrary, especially when the source of that polyunsaturated fat (so-called) is margarine, which has taken the place of butter in the butter dishes of more than two-thirds of all Americans.

Recent research points to margarine as a source of a substance which has been termed a far greater health risk than various cholesterol-containing supplements such as beef fat, butter fat, and powdered eggs, which it has supplanted in so many diets. **Dr. Fred Kummerow, a food chemist at the University of Illinois, says that this factor in margarine is causing atherosclerosis — the hardening of the arteries deemed the major triggering cause of coronary heart disease.**

Dr. Kummerow said that while margarine based on soybean oil is high in unsaturated fats in its original form, in actual commercial practice in the United States margarine producers utilize a process that converts a certain percentage of these fats — varying up to 30 per cent — to saturated forms. These converted fats, designed to make the product more stable, are called trans fats. **When Kummerow and his associates fed different types of diets to different groups of swine for eight months and then slaughtered them, they found that the trans fatty acids — margarine base stock — was more atherogenic than various cholesterol-containing substances like beef fat, butter and eggs.**

Even the highly touted polyunsaturated oils can be dangerous to health when they are heated, according to some very important research carried on at the Institute of Nutritional Chemistry at the University of Helsinki. Dr. Rakel Kurkela and his associates raised experimental animals on a standard diet, with a supplement of various fats, either in unheated native form or heated at a frying temperature for 20 hours. These fats were used in two different ways: heated and aerated (in an open dish, exposed to air as in frying) or heated and unaerated in a closed area (like baking). Fresh fats in the native state were also used.

The experiment lasted 10 to 30 days. Weight increases were measured daily. Those of the experimental animals on a diet supplement of butter had approximately the same weight gain whether the butter was heated and aerated or fed in a fresh unheated native state. In contrast, the animals which received unsaturated safflower oil in an unheated native state gained more weight than those raised on the butter. But, those animals receiving safflower oil which was heated and aerated had no weight gain at all. At the end of the 13 days of the experiment, all of the animals of this group were in poor condition. This shows, says Dr. Kurkela, that poisonous substances had formed during the aerating and heating of the oil. When these experiments were continued, all of the animals died.

How do you get the essential fats into your diet without lowering the boom on your chances for a healthy old age? Put the butter back in the butter dish. Natural butter, in moderation, is rich in vitamins A, D and E, which protect it from oxidation. To increase the butter's content of essential fatty acids, try this recipe for a modified butter: mix a half pound of softened butter with a half cup of a good pressed oil. Mold it in your butter dish and keep refrigerated. It tastes delicious. But for cooking, use the plain butter or olive oil. Raw seeds and nuts, freshly cracked, whole wheat and wheat germ are good sources of essential fatty acids. Make sure, though, that the wheat germ is fresh and not rancid.

If you have trouble digesting fats, you can get your essential fatty acids without eating them. Rub them into your skin. Dr. Martin Press and associates at the Royal Postgraduate Medical School at the Unilever Research Laboratory in Sharnbrook, Bedford, England, report that daily skin applications of sunflower seed oil rapidly corrected EFA deficiencies brought about by massive small bowel resections in three patients. In two of the patients, fatty acid patterns virtually returned to normal within 12 weeks. What's more, it took only two to three mg of linoleic acid per Kg to do the job. This, the researchers note, is at least 10 times less than any previous estimates of the amount required. When rubbed into the skin, they explain, linoleic acid is incorporated directly into circulating lipoproteins, bypassing the liver, where a great deal of it may be oxidized."

Editor: In the years since Dr. Ellis' passing in 1986, there have been many studies on the effects of dairy products in the diet. An extensive review article entitled *White Lies* that supports many of Dr. Ellis' opinions about milk and milk products is posted on the Viva! Health website at http://www.vegetarian.org.uk/campaigns/whitelies/wlreport02.shtml#vvf.

Milk and Milk Products

6 Detoxification

When you go to a doctor and are given a drug, a shot, or a prescription will it go into a cell that is filled with toxic material? You are just wasting your money. Get these toxins out of your system so your doctor has a chance to make an accurate diagnosis! Also, following detoxification, an individual's diagnosis will, in all probability, be entirely different from the admitting one!

Everything you eat and the way in that your body handles it depends on how toxic you are; i.e., whether your system needs to be detoxified. "Being toxic" means that the body is reabsorbing toxic materials from the digestive tract. Such materials include not only dyes and other chemicals but, more commonly, the products of inefficient digestive processes.

Digestion

There is a temporal order to the digestion of food, beginning in the mouth. The food must be chewed sufficiently. Most people attack their food and gulp the large particles rather than chew them properly. If the chewing action is complete, the bolus of food contains sufficient amounts of salivary enzymes and is alkaline so that it can trigger the stomach to produce hydrochloric acid.

The churning action of the stomach admixes hydrochloric acid into the food; the bolus now becomes acidic. This acidity triggers the flow of bile, which is highly alkaline. Bile neutralizes the hydrochloric acid as the bolus enters the small intestine, where the pancreatic secretions are favored by an alkaline environment. As the digested materials enter the large intestine, there is again encountered a more acidic environment where

Detoxification

---

bacterial flora further break down the foods and aid in the absorption of whatever products are formed at that stage.

Each successive step depends on the efficiency of the previous one. For the sake of illustration, let's assume that we eat only perfect quality foods in the proper combinations. Eating such good quality foods, how can one become toxic? Generally, by the time a person reaches his late teens or early twenties, he does not produce enough hydrochloric acid or pepsin in the stomach, especially if he has been bottle-fed.

The most important thing in your life is the colostrum in the first two hours after birth. These secretions help establish the way the digestive system will work all of the rest of your life. If you do not get these enzymes and bacteria, improper digestion will be a lifelong problem. In addition, we are in the habit of inadequately chewing our foods. The particles are too large by the time we swallow them, and this does not expose enough surface area for subsequent digestion. An insufficient amount of hydrochloric acid cannot provide enough acidity to induce bile secretion. Therefore, insufficient alkalinity for the optimum environment for pancreatic enzymes to work, etc. This leaves a herculean task for the acidophilus and bifidus bacilli to complete the digestive process. They simply cannot do as much as is required by inadequate digestion above the large intestine. Therefore, they produce undesirable breakdown products that are absorbed back into our bodies and that ruin the environment for the beneficial organisms. It becomes too toxic to support their growth. Inefficient breakdown of protein is termed putrefaction; inefficient breakdown of fats is called rancidification; inefficient breakdown of carbohydrates is termed fermentation. These are generally anaerobic processes that eventually produce an alkaline condition in the intestine with subsequent constipation and gas.

Resorption (reabsorption) of putrefied, rancidified, and fermented substances from the now sluggish bowel manifests itself in bad breath, body odor, and, as mentioned before, constipation. Other indications are a coated tongue, pasty skin, excessive bowel gas, too much oil on the skin, metallic or soapy taste, headaches behind the eyes, fatigue, and irritability. All of these symptoms are quite unnecessary, and the toxic condition should be avoided. Before one is able to sensibly attack any problem concerning health, he must ensure that he is detoxified! It is vitally important to remove the poisonous materials that develop from poor digestion and assimilation and correct your eating habits so that the food becomes available and usable.

Four Avenues of Detoxification

One thing that we have learned is that most people don't know how to detoxify themselves. **You must detoxify the body before you do anything else, because if it's filled with a lot of poisons and toxins, I don't care how many vitamins, minerals, enzymes or hormones, drugs or medicines you ingest; they can't get in. It's already full.** If they do try to get in, they can then push themselves out, and then we start seeing tumor formations. So that's something you definitely don't want to get into. So where do we start as far as detoxification is concerned?

We must understand the four avenues of detoxification — the lungs, the skin, the kidneys, and the bowel. Also, to some extent, the hair removes toxic minerals from the body. This post extension process is slow, however, and is a better indication of the presence of toxic metals than it is a way of eliminating such substances.

Lungs

The one that most people do not think about are the lungs. If you have a bad breath, it means you are constipated, because you're not getting the poisons out of your body any other way, so it's coming up through the lungs and out through the mouth. You can have infections as far as the teeth and the gums are concerned, but we find most bad body odors are caused by one thing — putrefied proteins. If you have a bad odor, but if it's not too bad, it is probably from fermented starch or sugar. Persons with bad breath (halitosis) are probably constipated. The use of Clorets can help eliminate the odor but does nothing to eliminate the cause. Remember these things. See Cleansing the Lungs on page 101.

Pores of the Skin

People do not like to have a body odor, so now they're doing something that is extremely harmful. They're using underarm antiperspirants, all of which block free perspiration, keeping the impurities from being excreted through the pores. All they're doing is stopping the flow of perspiration, keeping it in their bodies so they don't get rid of the poisons, and therefore they're going to break down.

Under no circumstances should you use an underarm antiperspirant. It is loaded with aluminum, which interferes with the circulation of every blood vessel in your body. We see this in the alteration of the ability of your body to take minerals from the bloodstream and get them into the cell to work properly. One thing that most people do not realize is that you urinate just as much as you perspire in one year. As you sit, you are perspiring. You may not realize it, but you are. That is why it is so necessary that we get enough fluids into our system to work on a daily basis. See Cleansing Through the Pores on page 101.

Kidneys

The third avenue that we have to think about is the kidneys. The kidneys must eliminate wastes and toxic products, but a tremendous strain is put on them in the toxic person. The kidneys are vital. That's why we do our standard types of urinalysis so we know what is going on. The microscopic portion of that is even more important than the actual amounts that tell you you might have a little albumin coming through with the ketones or the acetones, these are little things that we constantly look for. **Now any of you who may have any difficulty urinating, such as burning or itching after urination, it means one thing. You are too alkaline (the urine pH is too high).**

You see, all of these diseases in the genital urinary tract come when your body is too alkaline. Test the pH (that's your acid-alkaline balance) with a little litmus paper when you have these kinds of irritations; you will always find the pH to be above 7. A pH of 7 is neutral; normal should be on the acid side between 5 and 6. That is where we want to keep it. Here's another secret. If you have an itch anywhere on your body, you are too alkaline. It is very important to understand this. In all degenerative diseases that I have been able to find since I got into this research business, the people are too alkaline. See Cleansing the Kidneys on page 102.

Bowel

The big one, of course, is the bowel. The villi of the bowel must be clean with no materials or excessive mucous adhering to the bowel wall. These block absorption and elimination of wastes from the tissues into the bowel. **The most important thing is that you definitely have a bowel movement on a daily basis.**

An absolutely normal daily bowel movement is 1" in diameter, and it should be at least 18" long, whether you go once, twice or three times during the day. Now take a look at it; you should always take a look after you have had a bowel movement. If you don't have that one incher — if it starts getting smaller and smaller — what is it? You've got allergies. That causes the swelling of the mucous membranes in your rectum and up in your nose; the two ends of the tract is where you get it. That's where allergies hit you. See Cleansing the Bowel on page 102.

And where do you go from there? What causes it to shrink up? You see, when that fecal mass comes down and hits that swollen mucous membrane, you have a bunch of hemorrhoids. The other little thing I should tell you is don't read when you go to the toilet. You don't have any support down there and it all drops down and you have more hemorrhoids. When you have the urge to go, go in and get your business done; get off the hopper and get out of there in a hurry.

Cleansing the Lungs

Four steps are important to cleansing the lungs. First, put yourself in a private, healthy environment with clean air; then follow the steps as listed below.

1. Place the tip of the tongue at the base of the teeth, roof of mouth.
2. Breath in totally through the nose.
3. Let out 3/4 of the air with with an explosive HA! sound.
4. Without breathing in, expel more air with the HA! sound.
5. Again, without breathing in again, empty the lungs of the remaining air with a final, explosive HA! sound

Repeat this exercise as needed, several times during the day (without startling anyone)!

Cleansing Through the Pores

A sufficiently acidic pH in bath water can neutralize the charges around the pores of the skin and allow a free flow of substances in and out of the skin. To take advantage of this situation to cleanse through the pores, do the following.

1. Fill your bathtub with as hot a water as you can lie in.
2. Before getting in, carefully add two cups of household bleach (do not get the straight bleach on your skin or in your eyes or mouth).
3. Stir the water slowly for a few seconds to ensure that the bleach is diluted properly.
4. Get into the tub and lie in this mixture for 15-20 minutes.
5. Rinse off in a shower.

Take one such bath each day for seven days; the second week, every other day; the third week, every three days; then every four days; then every five days. When you are taking this bath once a week, remain on that schedule. If you begin to have problems with dry skin, discontinue the bath until your skin returns to normal and decrease the frequency of the bath.

Cleansing the Kidneys

Soluble toxins that are eliminated through the bowel are also eliminated through the kidneys. Basically, whatever works to detoxify the bowel will also detoxify the kidneys, but the high concentrations of these toxins can cause discomfort and damage. **What we are looking for is an acid pH of the urine, along with dilution of the toxins to minimize pain and harm to the kidney structures.**

Avoid milk and tap water, but **drink plenty of distilled water, adding apple cider vinegar to acidify the urine. Cranberry and black cherry juices help to create an acidic urine pH.** Avoid common over-the-counter pain killers and prescription drugs such as Librium and Valium. Millions of prescriptions are written in the United States for these; they are numbers one and two on the list of all prescribed items, and all they do is destroy your liver and your kidneys. Long-term use of pain killers also causes vascular disease.

Cleansing the Bowel

In the 5th century BC, Herodotus wrote: "The Egyptians clear themselves on three consecutive days, every month, seeking after health by emetics and enemas for they think that all disease comes to man from his food." So as you can see, the objective is to maintain a free flow of good quality foods and water through the body.

Deep breathing of fresh air, drinking of distilled water, frequent cleansing, and proper dietary habits are essential. A good habit to develop is to eat one or two tablespoons of raw, unprocessed bran daily. Be sure to drink plenty of water with it; otherwise, constipation could set in. **Do not use the cereal forms of bran**; these have been infiltrated with sugar and other chemicals.

Now, if you are not feeling good or, for example, if you feel as though a cold is coming on, don't wait for it to get there. Catch it! That's why I say we predict life. Don't wait until you get sicker; we want to predict what is going to happen to you if you don't take care of yourself. So you're going to have to think, "How am I going to detoxify myself to get all of this out of me?" Several digestive tract detoxification procedures are outlined below.

Vigorous Laxative

A laxative taken by mouth is sometimes called a physic. Take two tablespoons of Fleet's Phospho-Soda in a glass of cold water. Follow this with a glass of hot water. This flushes the gallbladder and liver; the bile activates the bowel within 15 minutes to two hours. If the constipation is severe, it may take a dose every two hours, up to a maximum of three doses, until you get results.

While you are waiting for the laxative to take effect, take a lemon juice enema. It is prepared by putting the juice of a freshly-squeezed and strained lemon into two quarts of warm water. This solution will dissolve excess mucous in the bowel. Use the recommended enema technique described below.

Mild Laxative

Drink a quarter cup of aloe vera gel (not the juice) twice a day. If constipation is severe, the gel can be taken in prune, cranberry, or apple juice. What aloe vera does by mouth is empty the gallbladder and the liver to bring out the poisonous material. The bile activates the intestinal tract in a normal way, and the aloe vera helps to heal as it's going through.

The desirable reaction is a liquid stool for 10 days. If this is not obtained, use three or four ounces twice a day. Taper off to a loose but formed stool by reducing the morning amount by 1/3 every three days. Once you have the cleansing effect, keep at it. If there are food allergies, the digestive membranes will be swelled. The aloe vera gel will help heal these and reduce the swelling.

Detoxification

Herbal Laxatives

Not being an expert on herbs, I will not comment on their use. There are some good herbal cleansing remedies, but they should not be used indefinitely. Consult a competent herbalist.

> **Editor:** For information, see the website of Dr. John Christopher at http://www.drchristopher.com/.

Recommended Enema Technique

Developed all of the way back In 1931, during my internship at the hospital, the proper technique in taking a cleansing or retention enema is as follows. Lie flat on your back. Make sure that the enema bag is never higher than 12" above your abdomen, preferably 10".

Cleansing Enema

For a cleansing enema, take two quarts in never less that 20 minutes, preferably 30 minutes. The slower the better. If you hit a fecal impaction or a gas pocket, it'll dilate the bowel and cause pain. When you do that always just grab hold of the tube and squeeze it and just hold onto it while the peristaltic activity works on that fecal impaction. Or if it's a gas pocket, you will find all of a sudden the peristaltic action will move it, and you will hear the gurgling as the water comes in, the pressure goes off, the pain goes out, then you can continue it until you get the whole two quarts in. If you do it that slowly then you can hang up the enema bag, and walk around for five minutes before you have to expel it.

Do not use the inferior Fredger enema cleansing enema technique, where you put it in and hold the bag up as high as you can. All that happens is a rectal dilatation, but you never get an enema. It never gets cleansing up into the colon. And when you get done and let the water out, the pressure is so great you can't hold it in.

You see, the higher you put the bag and the more force you use in an enema, the more you dilate the rectum and throw it into spasm. Actually, a person can hold three quarts, so two is not too much to ask for. If it hits a fecal impaction or a gas pocket, you immediately get the dilatation of the colon and it produces pain. If it does, pinch the tube, wait until the peristaltic action goes to work on it, and the first thing you know, it loosens up, the pressure comes down, the rest of the water goes in very easily, and you can release the pressure on the tube to let the rest of the water get in there. If you have done it slowly enough, you don't have any pain so you can get up and walk around a bit. Then sit down on the toilet and expel it. That is the proper method of taking an enema.

Retention Enema

For a retention enema, the amount we use is usually one pint. The idea with a retention enema is to keep it inside the digestive tract as long as it's possible. In other words, if you can absorb a whole pint, that's great. If you can't and it finally gets to where the peristaltic activity is pushing it down into the rectal fossa to where you get the reflex, then you better get on the toilet quickly and get rid of what is left unabsorbed. It is appropriate to take a cleansing enema first and then take a retention enema. One can make an enema out of any of the following mixtures.

Aloe Vera Cleansing Enema

We try to start patients off in the morning, usually with the aloe vera gel enema to get the bowel open; we use it most of the time. They have pretty good bowel movements, and we get an acceptable level of cleanliness. Then we follow it up with a vitamin C or coffee enema. We've tested about 15 different companies and found Lily of the Desert to be the best gel.

Preparation

The mixture is four to eight ounces of aloe vera gel diluted with water to a total of two quarts.

Technique

Use the recommended cleansing enema technique, as described above. Our bowels are shaped with villi on the inside. If you have anything stuck in between the villi, you can have three bowel movements a day and still be constipated. Aloe vera helps to grease the track as it goes down, and therefore allows the normal enzymatic activity of each of these villi, with their digestive enzymes, to digest the food. Therefore it allows the food to come through in a normal and natural way with no problems. If hemorrhoids are present or the rectum is otherwise inflamed, put two ounces of the gel in a baby syringe and administer it rectally at bedtime. Retain this material overnight.

Vitamin C Retention Enema

Any degenerative disease state needs a lot of vitamin C. Cancer, diabetes, arthritis — all of them are related to one another; there's only a little variance in the cell chemistry and in what you have to do to get them straightened out. We're finding on the arthritics we're treating some excellent results by giving two and three of these vitamin C enemas on a daily basis.

Preparation

Make a solution of 4,000 mg of ascorbic acid to one pint of water.

Technique

Again we use the recommended technique. This is not a cleansing enema, but a way of infusing a large amount of vitamin C into the system. Retain this solution so as much of it can be absorbed as possible. Many persons experience a shift from alkaline to acid urine; this is desirable. Taking the amounts of vitamin C recommended by Pauling (50-60 gm daily) by mouth may not be practical. Using the enema form of administration, one may take as much as 10 gm.

Coffee Retention Enema

The coffee enema was popularized by Dr. Max Gerson in his work on cancer. However, it is now used in association with a wide variety of degenerative disease conditions. Coffee is something that we put in the wrong end. You have no business putting it in your mouth, it should only be used for enemas. Coffee by mouth is a diuretic; it is hard on the kidneys and helps to deplete the body of potassium and the B complex vitamins. Actually, the toxic material in coffee is the oil. As mentioned above, oils and fats are subject to rancidification. This occurs quickly after the beans are roasted and ground, and these rancid oils upset the liver and kidneys.

Preparation

The proper technique in the use of coffee enemas is to start with unground coffee beans. When you grind the coffee beans, the oil that's in the coffee bean immediately starts turning rancid. So when you make coffee and add more heat to it, you make it more rancid. When you drink it, the rancidity of that coffee oil is very detrimental to you.

Take a tablespoon of coffee beans to a cup and a half of water. Do a slow boil for 10 minutes; in other words don't put the flame up real high, just a low flame, just so you see it boiling for 10 minutes. Then drain the liquid off of the coffee beans so you only have the liquid coffee. Then you add to that (it's usually that cup and a half that'll boil down to a half a cupful, so you end up with about one cup). Add three cups of warm water to it and then take your coffee enema.

Technique

Again use the recommended technique, but with a retention enema. This is not a cleansing enema. What it does is provide caffeine to stimulate the emptying of the gallbladder and the liver and help you detoxify yourself. It also stimulates the adrenal glands and the setting up of your cortisone preparations. They are your anti-inflammatory agents, and that's what the coffee enemas are for. In the coffee work of Dr. Gerson, you are asked to take five of these every day so you're running about every three hours to take one as long as you possibly can.

We have developed one that I think is working better today. We have found that, if we alternate using 8,000 mg of ascorbic acid to a pint of water with the coffee enemas every three hours — first coffee, then the vitamin C, then coffee, vitamin C, coffee. By using it in this method, we are today getting better results in detoxifying and stimulating the cancer people. It brings them out of it faster than any other way we know. It does beautiful work.

Other Supplements

You can make a solution of the desired number of units of vitamin A, vitamin E, coenzyme Q, or any other water- or oil-soluble vitamin preparation in one pint of water and administer them in a retention enema. This is a way of infusing these substances directly into the system. Retain this solution so as much of it can be absorbed as possible.

Fasting (Not Eating)

I am not a believer in any form of fasting. I am one who is a great disbeliever in our day and age that fasting should be used. I have seen too many of my friends die of congestive heart failure as the result of a 12-day fast!

When I talk to a lot of these people who are great believers in fasting, most of them have the same idea that the object is to change their alkaline bodies to an acid and head them in that direction and this is why we run into all of these problems, charley horses in a heart muscle, for instance, that kills you. **Consequently, if you must fast, I recommend that you go to an institution that is familiar with fasting. Do it under supervision; do not do it at home.**

Fasting Alternative (Quick Grapefruit Fast)

Because of the dangers of fasting, we decided to develop some methods to offset the risks. We devised an alternative method that is equal to a 12-day fast; we do it all in one day. **It is what I call a one-day grapefruit fast.** Buy sixteen (16) grapefruit and a bottle of betaine-HCl and pepsin tablets. Peel the grapefruit and leave the white on it; that is where the bioflavonoids are contained. Eat four grapefruit (everything but the seeds) and take three of the betaine-HCl and pepsin tablets four times during the day (8:00 AM, 12:00 noon, 4:00 PM, and lastly at 8:00 PM). This is your entire diet for the day (16 grapefruit and 12 betaine hydrochloride and pepsin tablets), and you had better drink plenty of water! The more toxic you are, the more strongly will adverse reactions set in.

Usually about 3:00 PM you're not sure you want to look another grapefruit in the eye because it's going to start pulling the poison out of your system so much that you're going to start feeling so toxic that you just don't feel like trying to eat another one of those grapefruit. At this particular time, take a lemon enema to clean yourself out. When you do that, it will be simple to eat the four grapefruit at 4:00 PM in the afternoon and again at 8:00 PM that night.

At about 9:00 PM, you will feel very bad. However, this is to be expected and should simply be tolerated; the bad feelings will pass. Another lemon enema will aid in getting the toxins out of the body more quickly. But believe you me that cleans you out. We have a lot of families today that are doing this one Sunday a month; the whole family gets into it. We do this even on hypoglycemics, the worst type. We've done it on diabetics. We have no problems with it, but on these we would rather use the slow aloe vera gel method.

For additional nutrition, take a teaspoon and just peel the white out of the peel and eat it. That's where the rest of the bioflavonoids are; that's part of your natural vitamin C complex, called civatemic acid. It is made up of ascorbogen from which ascorbic acid comes. Bioflavonoids, folic acid, rutin, and vitamin K are part of this C complex. When we use anything like ascorbic acid or sodium ascorbate, we always use a tablet of the natural C complex to get the catalytic activity of the natural synergistic factors to make the ascorbic acid or the sodium ascorbate work.

By the end of a day of eating the pulp of the grapefruit, the teeth may become sensitive. This is found in some patients, especially if they are too low in calcium. If this is the case, you must be careful of citrus; the older you get the less oranges you want to eat. All oranges are picked green and dyed to make you think they are ripe but they are not.

Fasting Alternative (Slow Aloe Vera Method)

The slow method involves the use of aloe vera gel. We prefer Lily of the Desert brand. This method is the easy one. For 10 days we want a liquid stool, so we have the patient drink two ounces (a quarter cup) of aloe vera gel morning and night. This type of gel is thick, like gelatin just before it gets a little hard. That's the way it comes in the bottle. If you have a little trouble swallowing it, add a little cranberry juice or apple juice to it, then you will have no problem.

If two ounces isn't enough twice a day to get that liquid stool, take three or four ounces. In other words, build up to a half a cup twice a day because we want that liquid stool for 10 days. If you're so toxic and so loaded with poison that the half a cup twice a day does not give you a liquid stool, then you had better take a good dose of castor oil and really flush yourself out. Then go back to the two ounces of the aloe vera morning and night.

After 10 days of the liquid stool, cut it back to where you have a loose but a formed stool. Cut out 1/3 of whatever the amount is that you take on the morning dose first, every three days, so at the end of nine days, you're finished with the one in the evening. You might bring it down to where you're only taking a teaspoonful; you never know, every person is different. We have some people that have to take two ounces morning and night just to have the loose but formed stool because we are that much different in our individuality. But whatever the amount is to get that loose but formed stool, that is the amount we want you to stay on for never less than three months. That's the slow time, all of the way through.

I have taken this for as much as 16 consecutive months just to find out, because I have heard of so many detrimental things if you continue to take it over a long period of time. I saw no detrimental effects whatsoever as far as my own health was concerned, because I'm pretty sensitive to such things.

Colonic Irrigation

A lot of people don't understand what a colonic irrigation is. It is a glorified enema. Instead of using two quarts of water, you use from five to 30 gallons of water. But you want to be very careful where you go to have colonic irrigations. **They are absolutely the finest therapy I know for high blood pressure; with colonic irrigations, you don't need anything else. To me a Dierker Colonic is, by far, the ideal one.** I do not like gravitational types because you have to depend upon a sick bowel to tell you how much pressure you have before you try to expel it.

> **Editor:** The Dierker closed system colonic machine is no longer being manufactured under that name. Some used units are available on the internet. The reader may refer to the International Association for Colon Hydrotherapy publication, *Colon Therapy, 2 Edition*, found at https://www.cga.ct.gov/2013/phdata/tmy/2013SB-00873-R000220-International%20Assoc%20for%20Colon%20Therapy%20(I-ACT)-TMY.PDF.

No Detoxification is Complete Without This!

So many people have indecisions, fears, anxieties, irritabilities. and tensions. The worst one of all to get out of the system is hatred. If you project these things through a negative attitude toward people, you get back with interest what you give!

Look for the good in everything, no matter how bad it may seem at the moment; because when you go back and realize what had happened to you years later, you will find out that it was the finest thing that ever happened to you. If you keep in a positive realm within the mind, you will be able to accept the next opportunity that comes along.

What you must do more than any one thing is to start projecting love! If you still have a negative mind, you are going to miss all those opportunities. You're not going to get anywhere. The one thing that you have to do to get rid of all of these negative factors, and especially hatred, is in the spoken word, not in actions. For instance, if you husbands didn't say "I love you" to your wives when you got up this morning, if you wives didn't say "I love you" to your husbands, if you parents didn't say "I love you" to their children and if your children haven't been taught to say "I love you", you have started your day wrong.

One of the hardest things I find with people is to get out this spoken word — to talk and give love to other people. The Bible taught me to love my neighbor as myself. I'm going to start you on the right road now. When you encounter someone, shake his or her hand and say, "God loves you, and so do I!" That's your detoxification plan in a hurry!

Detoxification

7   Nutritional Supplements

Today, because of processing, bleaching, and canning of foods, we find very few foods that are of top quality and contain all of the nutrients that a person (especially one with vicarious eating habits) needs on a regular basis.

Although it is possible to get all of the vitamins, minerals, and protein that you need from a perfect diet of natural, high-quality foods, very few people are ever able to maintain such a diet. Therefore, it is usually necessary to take supplements to make up for the lack of food quality. See Food Supplements on page 225.

It is also possible to overdo supplementation. Some doctors prescribe from 400 to 800 vitamin and mineral pills a day. They are overstimulating their patients to the point of inhibition. They are getting some symptomatic changes in the patient where they might feel better for a while, but they usually end up in trouble later on. That's not what we want.

Let's talk about various nutritional supplements to the diet and how they are used, limiting the types to the following.

- Vitamins
- Minerals
- Emulsified Vitamins and Coenzymes
- Digestives
- Glandulars (Protomorphogens)
- Adjuncts
- Herbs

Vitamins

A vitamin is an organic (carbon-containing) compound essential for normal growth and good health. They may be fat- or water-soluble and are required in small quantities in the diet, because they are not synthesized by the body in sufficient amounts. Rather, they are synthesized by bacteria in the digestive system and contained in foods. Vitamins act as coenzymes that regulate metabolic processes but do not provide energy (as do sugars and fats) or building blocks (as do proteins). Deficiencies of vitamins produce specific disorders.

Everyone has what Dr. Roger Williams of the University of Texas calls *biochemical individuality.* That means that there is a world of difference between you and, say, your brother or sister. You may need twice the quantity of one nutrient, yet less than half the quantity of another, compared to your relatives. This is not theory; it is fact. **No one can set a maximum or minimum daily requirement of any nutrient. To do so is to thoroughly ignore the principle of biochemical individuality.**

Fat-soluble Vitamins

Fat-soluble vitamins require dietary fat to facilitate absorption. They are stored in the liver and in body fat and used as needed. Ingesting more fat-soluble vitamins than you need can be toxic, causing side-effects like nausea, vomiting, and liver and heart problems. These include those listed in Table 4, with actions and dietary sources indicated.

Table 4: Fat-soluble Vitamins

Name	Actions	Dietary Sources	Comments
Vitamin A (Retinol, Retinal, Retinoic Provitamin A, Carotenoids)	Antioxidant, benefits the eyes and vision, the development of bones, and aids immune functions.	Dark-colored fruits and vegetables; dark leafy greens, fish liver oil, egg yolk, butter, liver, beef, and fish	Synthesized in the body from carotenes present in the diet.
Vitamin D (Dihydrotachysterol, Calcitriol, or Ergocalciferol)	Offsets skeletal disease through promotion of calcium absorption.	Fish liver oils and sunlight	A severe vitamin D deficiency can cause muscle weakness and pain.
Vitamin E (Alpha-tocopherol)	Antioxidant, protecting cells from free radicals formed during energy metabolism.	Cereals, leafy green vegetables, seeds, and nuts, avocado, dark green vegetables, oils wheat germ	An excess may cause muscle weakness and gastrointestinal disorders.
Vitamin K (Koagulationsvitamin)	Coagulant, active in preventing coronary artery disease, osteoporosis, possibly valuable in offsetting dementia.	Dark green leafy vegetables, cabbage, cauliflower, cereals, fish, liver, beef, and eggs	Synthesized by intestinal bacteria

With the emulsions of both vitamin A, and E, you get more activity than with the non-emulsified types. So, you use these in very small amounts. The vitamin E that we use is 35 units. You would use only about three drops a day. You get 300 times the activity as you would with any other vitamin so you don't have to take too much of it.

Water-soluble Vitamins

Water-soluble vitamins are not stored in your body and must be replenished daily. Your body takes what it needs from the food you eat and then excretes what is not needed as waste. All B vitamins help the body convert carbohydrates into glucose, which the body uses to produce energy. These B vitamins, often referred to as B-complex vitamins, also help the body metabolize fats and protein.

Editor: Dr. Ellis did not customarily use individual vitamins and minerals for their singular pharmacological effects in treating specific conditions. Rather, he used them in what he believed was an appropriate combination to support the general health of an individual patient under his care. For more information, refer to the WebMD website: http:// www.webmd.com/drugs/index-drugs.aspx.

The water-soluble vitamins are listed in Table 5, with some actions and dietary sources indicated.

Table 5:   Water-soluble Vitamins

Name	Actions	Dietary Sources	Comments
Vitamin B1 (Thiamin)	Offsets conditions such as Beriberi, lung congestion, heart failure, burning of the toes and feet, leg cramps, and muscle wasting.	Whole grains, liver, nuts, seeds, eggs, lean meats, legumes, beans, organ meats, peas, whole grains	When too much B1 is taken by itself, it becomes toxic to the human body, causing headache, insomnia, irritability, contact dermatitis.
Vitamin B2 (Riboflavin, old term: Vitamin G)	Offsets conditions such as jaundice, anemia, anorexia/ bulimia, cataracts, loss of cognitive function, depression, migraines, weakness, sore throat and tongue, cracks in the corners of the mouth, blurred vision, and light sensitivity.	Whole grains, enriched grains, and dairy products (not allowed in the Ellis plan)	Most people in a stress pattern are highly nervous and irritable, so we use vitamin B2. It is destroyed by sunlight.

Doctor to Patient

Name	Actions	Dietary Sources	Comments
Vitamin B3 (Niacin, Niacinamide)	Niacin is commonly used as a vasodilator. Offsets high cholesterol. Because of its vasodilating ability, it is used in combination with other modalities for treating a variety of conditions.	Meat, fish, poultry, whole grains, avocado, eggs, fish (tuna and salt-water fish), lean meats, legumes, nuts, potatoes, poultry	An excess can cause liver damage and skin irritation. It is synthesized in the body from tryptophan.
Vitamin B5 (Pantothenic Acid)	Offsets osteoarthritis, acne, alcoholism, allergies, and a host of other conditions too numerous to mention here. Gives protection against mental and physical stress and anxiety. It is applied topically for itching skin.	Meat, poultry, whole grains, avocado, vegetables in the cabbage family, eggs, legumes, lentils, mushrooms, organ meats, poultry, white and sweet potatoes	Large daily doses of pantothenic acid can cause swelling of the ankles, wrists and face, with itching and local sensitivity, depression, and joint pain.
Vitamin B6 (Pyridoxine)	Pyridoxine is needed for normal brain development and function, and helps the body make the hormones serotonin and norepinephrine.	Soy products, avocado, banana, legumes, beans, meat, nuts, poultry, whole grains	An excess may cause peripheral nerve damage. Requirement is related to protein intake.

Name	Actions	Dietary Sources	Comments
Vitamin B7 (Biotin)	Biotin is used to support adrenal function, to help calm and maintain a healthy nervous system. Offsets hair loss, fatigue, depression, nausea, muscle pains, and anemia.	Cereal, egg yolk, legumes, nuts, organ meats (liver, kidney), pork, yeast	High levels of pantothenic acid, some anti-seizure drugs, and smoking can affect the levels of biotin.
Vitamin B9 (Folic Acid)	Folic acid is important for the production and maintenance of new cells, prevention of anemia, proper brain function and mental and emotional health.	Leafy vegetables, asparagus, broccoli, beets, yeast, beans (cooked pinto, navy, kidney, and lima), lentils, oranges, wheat germ	It can mask a deficiency of B12.
Vitamin B12 (Cyanocobal-amin)	Vitamin B12 helps in making DNA and red blood cells. Offsets the effects of a dam-aged stomach lining, perni-cious anemia, Chron's disease, celiac disease, and long-term use of acid-reducing drugs.	Fish, poultry, meat, eggs, organ meats (liver and kid-ney), shellfish	Absorption requires intrinsic factor produced by the stomach. It is found only in foods of animal origin, so strict vegetarians and vegans must take supplements.

Doctor to Patient

Nutritional Supplements

Name	Actions	Dietary Sources	Comments
Vitamin C (Ascorbic Acid)	Ascorbic acid is a powerful antioxidant that fights free radicals. It helps the body form and repair numerous tissues in the body.	Citrus fruit (tree-ripened), such as oranges and grapefruits; red, yellow, and green peppers, broccoli, brussels sprouts, cabbage, cauliflower, potatoes, spinach, strawberries, tomatoes	Can cause diarrhea and oxalate kidney stones. It can be destroyed by cooking in the presence of air and plant enzymes released by cutting and grating. Watch for inflammation of the intestine. Drink plenty of water.

I use natural vitamin C complex 4,000 mg (a teaspoonful) four times a day, at each meal and at bedtime. If taken by mouth, always take the natural vitamin C complex for each 1,000 mg of ascorbic acid or sodium ascorbate. Of course, other factors in the formation of arteriosclerosis and atherosclerosis must be taken into consideration. Vitamin C is an oxidizer and an acidifier, and one of the reasons people get diarrhea from taking ascorbic acid by mouth is that they were so highly alkaline when they took an extra amount of the ascorbic acid — the acid factor. They get a big change in body chemistry. That's what creates dehydration, pulling the fluid into the bowel. You can clear up more diarrheas by taking a physic and an enema than any other method that I know of.

Fillers

Many companies use starches and sugars for their fillers. These detract from or may even neutralize the effectiveness of the supplement. Biotics Research Corporation uses sprouts — peas and lentils. To the liquid used in sprouting, they add certain vitamins and minerals, which are then incorporated into the sprouts. After several days, the sprouts are dehydrated at 89° F, ground up, and used as fillers for their tablets. The catalyst effect is fantastic, and we get better results using their products.

Minerals

Minerals are nutrients found in the earth or water; they are absorbed by plants and animals for proper nutrition. Minerals are the main component of teeth and bones and help build cells and support nerve impulses, among other things. Minerals are customarily classified into two groups, nutritional (macrominerals and trace minerals) and toxic. Every mineral in large excess is toxic, but those in the toxic group have virtually no effect except toxicity.

Minerals are vital, because they make the enzymes in every cell and every function that takes place within your body. So if you don't have those minerals in their proper ratios to one another, they'll never work. Vitamins are the catalysts that make the minerals become enzyme systems, so if you don't have those balanced properly, it is impossible for them to become enzymes. There is only one-quarter ounce of vitamins in a 160-pound person, but it is the ratios of these, one to the other, that make all of these coordinate into a healthy individual.

Sometimes, a mineral level is fairly closely related to current dietary behavior, such as the scarcity of zinc, which is seen commonly in vegetarians. Sometimes, the influence is roundabout, such as the tendency of people who do not get enough of the vitamin B complex to develop scarcities of sodium and potassium. Some tissue minerals are high when the body is losing them or transporting them to another location, such as the excess seen in osteoporosis. Some minerals interfere with other minerals, such as excessive selenium causing a scarcity of copper.

The subject of minerals is one vitally important to each of us. Let's lay some groundwork. Each of the minerals we require is equally capable of combining in the digestive tract with some other material to form an inassimilable compound. Even calcium can combine with phytates from whole grains or oxalic acid from spinach to form compounds that the body cannot use. **Consequently, mineral nutrition is never just a simple matter of numbers.** For instance, if we lack chromium we may not notice the lack for many years until we develop maturity onset diabetes. A good book on mineral metabolism is *The Trace Elements and Man* by Henry A. Schroeder, M.D.

It is important to know exactly which amino acid is best suited for a particular mineral and how to chelate it exactly as nature does it. Anything less than natural will also be less than ideal for the purpose. That is why certain companies come out on top with all of their products. Especially good is Miller Pharmaceutical Co.; also good is Biotics Research Corporation. So when dealing with minerals, be aware of all of these facts.

How to Take and Not Take Minerals

It is important to learn how the minerals blend (not interfere) with each other, so you can get them into your body without wasting them. There's no testing method that we know of to determine this. Depending on what we find in a hair mineral analysis and bloodwork, along with knowing what the ratios are to one another, we can determine which minerals to give someone and when to take them. Certain minerals, we have found, have no best time to take or not take, such as potassium. **Do not try to take all of your minerals at the same time, such as are found in dolomite. Dolomite is loaded with aluminium and lead to very high toxic amounts.**

Mineral Summaries

The following tables list information about various minerals. Macrominerals (Table 6) and trace minerals (Table 7) are important and beneficial to body functions and should be taken, when necessary, to supplement deficiencies. Toxic metals (Table 8 and Table 9) are dangerous to body functions and should be avoided. The toxic metals are listed in this chapter to help the reader understand possible interactions with the beneficial minerals.

Table 6: Summary of Macrominerals

Macrominerals	
Name	**Notes**
Calcium	**Take upon waking on an empty stomach with betaine hydrochloride or acidic juices (cranberry or black cherry). Do not take at the same time as magnesium or manganese.** Calcium is absorbed from the upper parts of the small intestine. The amount of absorption depends on the acidity of the intestinal contents and the amount of phosphate present. Calcium salts are soluble in acids. Calcium, along with protein, phosphorus, and magnesium are important to the formation of bone. The remaining 1% of the calcium in the body is essential for blood clotting, blood pressure stabilization, normal brain function, glucose metabolism, and contraction of muscles.
Magnesium	**Take at suppertime. Do not take at the same time as calcium.** Magnesium is needed for more than 300 biochemical reactions in the body. It helps to maintain normal nerve and muscle function, supports a healthy immune system, keeps the heart beat steady, and helps bones remain strong. It also helps to regulate blood glucose levels and aid in the production of energy and protein. One can for a long time be nervous, irritable, or easily fatigued with no awareness of a deficiency of magnesium and potassium. Magnesium is commonly administered as a sulfate; but the absorption is 2.6 times as great when in the amino acid chelated form.

Nutritional Supplements

Macrominerals	
Name	Notes
Phosphorus	**Take half way between breakfast and lunch and lunch and supper and sometimes as an aid to digesting carbohydrates. Do not take at the same time as calcium.** Phosphorus is a major component of bone, but it also combines with lipids to make phospholipids, a major structural component of all cell membranes, or walls, throughout the body. Phospholipids in brain cells control which minerals, nutrients and drugs go in and out of the cell. Phosphorus is required for energy production and storage, helping the body change protein, fat, and carbohydrate into energy. As a component of DNA and RNA, phosphorus is also involved in the storage and transmission of genetic material. It activates enzymes, hormones, and cell-signaling molecules through phosphorylation. Phosphorus also helps to get oxygen to tissues and buffers a normal pH.
Potassium	**Take at no particular time.** Potassium, along with sodium, maintain heartbeat and nerve function. They also regulate hydration in accordance with the adrenal hormone, aldosterone. The potassium level rises from kidney disease, use of diuretics, and the use of aldosterone supplements, causing muscle weakness, tingling, and even cardiac arrest. A potassium deficiency is more common, with similar symptoms to that of an elevated level, such as kidney malfunction, vomiting, and dangerous heart arrhythmias. Along with a supplement, eat ripe bananas, avocados, and parsley.
Sodium	**Provided by salt-containing foods.** Sodium and potassium are electrolytes that work together to carry electrical charges in the body, facilitating muscle contraction and nerve cell transmission. They maintain normal water balance in the body, thereby keeping control of the body's blood volume and blood pressure. If either blood volume or sodium levels get too high, the kidneys are stimulated to excrete excess sodium, returning blood volume to normal levels. It is recommend that people limit sodium intake to 2,400 mg, but most Americans consume 4,000–6,000 mg a day.

Macrominerals	
Name	**Notes**
Sulfur	**Usually provided by a protein source.** Sulfur is a component of four amino acids: methionine, cysteine, cystine, and taurine and is highly concentrated in the protein structure of the joints, hair, nails, and skin. It is also important in the production of insulin, which is rich in sulfur-containing amino acids. Certain conditions, such as arthritis and liver disorders, may be improved by increasing the intake of sulfur, which is found in good quantity in sulfur-rich foods, such as eggs, legumes, whole grains, garlic, onions, brussel sprouts, and cabbage. Deficiencies occur only with a severe lack of protein.

Table 7: Summary of Trace Minerals

Trace Minerals	
Name	**Notes**
Boron	Arthritis and osteoporosis are managed by using boron, and it helps to relieve menopausal symptoms. It is believed to improve the body's ability to absorb calcium and magnesium. Boron is used for building strong bones and muscles, increasing testosterone levels, and improving thinking and muscle coordination. Boric acid is used to kill yeast that cause vaginal infections.
Chromium	Chromium helps insulin transport glucose into cells, where it can be used for energy. Chromium also appears to be involved in the metabolism of carbohydrate, fat, and protein. It may play a role in the management of type 2 diabetes. Low chromium levels may be associated with increased risk of glaucoma. Chromium slows the loss of calcium, so it may help prevent bone loss. Chromium has a toxic form that is chemically different from its nutritional form. If the measured level of chromium is low, there is a scarcity (not necessarily a deficiency) of the nutritional form. If the level is high, there may be an excess of either form.
Cobalt	Although commonly used in electroplating and the production of alloys, cobalt is an essential trace dietary mineral for all animals, being the active center of coenzymes called cobalamins, the most common example of which is vitamin B12. Cobalt is beneficial to the circulatory system, and, along with iodine and copper, improves light sensitivity, reducing glare, and improving vision.
Copper	Copper has 5.8 times better absorption as an amino acid chelate (5.8 times as much as copper carbonate, 3 times as much as copper oxide, and 4.1 times as much as copper sulfate). Copper is essential as a trace dietary mineral because it is a constituent of the respiratory enzyme complex cytochrome c oxidase. In humans, copper is found mainly in the liver, muscle, and bone.

Trace Minerals	
Name	**Notes**
Germanium	We have noticed that germanium promotes more efficient use of oxygen in the body. The main effect of germanium is to increase the oxidative index of blood and body. Studies on germanium therapy for cancer were done by Dr. Asai in northern Japan. Germanium can easily cure blue lips. The lips start to get pinker and pinker. Other food sources of germanium are ginseng and garlic; they are both very high. Garlic caps from Japan are most effective. Take them 30 minutes before meal.
Iodine	Iodine is not only required for proper function of the thyroid, other tissues absorb and use large amounts of iodine, including the breasts, salivary glands, pancreas, cerebral spinal fluid, skin, stomach, brain, and thymus gland. Iodine deficiency in any of these tissues may cause dysfunction of that tissue.

Take only a few drops in juice. Take care not to overdose; there are many recommendations about dosage, but one indicator of excessive intake is development of a sore throat, independent of a cold or other infection.

The following symptoms may point to insufficient intake of iodine in the diet: dry mouth, dry skin, lack of perspiration, reduced alertness, nodules or scars in the muscles, along with pain, such as fibrosis or fibromyalgia.

Editor: See the article *The Silent Epidemic of Iodine Deficiency*. October 2011, by Nancy Piccone at http://www.lifeextension.com/magazine/2011/10/the-silent-epidemic-of-iodine-deficiency/Page-01. |

Nutritional Supplements

Trace Minerals	
Name	**Notes**
Iron	Iron gives black stools when it is not absorbed; it also causes constipation. If properly chelated; you never see black stool or constipation. **It is best to take iron tablets before bed**; you will have more absorption and the stomach will be less irritable at that time. Avoid taking vitamin E with iron, as they neutralize and are not absorbed. (If the stool is black and tarry; blood is present; if it is black with its usual consistency, iron is usually present).
Lithium	Commonly used for its mood altering pharmacological effects. Lithium is used to treat manic depression with its hyperactivity, poor judgment, sleep deprivation, aggression, and anger.
Manganese	Manganese is found mostly in the bones, liver, kidneys, and pancreas and helps the body form connective tissue, bones, blood clotting factors, and sex hormones. It also plays a role in fat and carbohydrate metabolism, calcium absorption, and blood sugar regulation. Manganese is also necessary for normal brain and nerve function. It is a cofactor of the antioxidant enzyme superoxide dismutase (SOD), which fights free radicals. Low levels of manganese in the body can contribute to infertility, bone malformation, weakness, and seizures. Too much manganese in the diet could lead to neurological disorders or poor cognitive performance. A proper level of manganese may offset osteoporosis, arthritis, PMS, diabetes, and epilepsy. **Take at lunchtime. Do not take at the same time as calcium.** Dietary sources of manganese include nuts and seeds, wheat germ and whole grains (including unrefined cereals, buckwheat, bulgur wheat, and oats), legumes, and pineapples.

Trace Minerals	
Name	**Notes**
Molybdenum	Molybdenum deficiency results in high blood levels of sulfite and urate. Dietary molybdenum deficiency from low soil concentration of molybdenum has been associated with increased rates of esophageal cancer in China and Iran. Because it is an antagonist of copper, molybdenum can prevent plasma proteins from binding to copper, increasing the amount of copper excreted in urine. A congenital molybdenum cofactor deficiency disease, seen in infants, results in interference with the ability of the body to use molybdenum in enzymes. It causes high levels of sulfite and urate, and neurological damage.
Rubidium	Rubidium has no known biological role and is non-toxic. However, because it is chemically similar to potassium, we absorb it from our food, and the average person stores about 1/2 gm.
Selenium	Commonly used in the glass and photocell industries, selenium is involved in some health conditions — such as HIV, Crohn's disease, and others that are associated with low selenium levels. People fed intravenously are also at risk for low selenium.

Doctor to Patient

Nutritional Supplements

Trace Minerals	
Name	**Notes**
Vanadium	Vanadium is used to make alloys for jet engines, in bonding titanium to steel, and with gallium to form superconducting magnets. Vanadium pentoxide is used in ceramics and as a catalyst for the production of sulfuric acid. In the body, vanadium is used to treat diabetes, low blood sugar, high cholesterol, heart disease, tuberculosis, syphilis, a form of tired blood (anemia), and water retention (edema). It is also used for improving athletic performance in weight training and for preventing cancer.
Zinc	**Take before or with a meal, depending on need. Do not take on an empty stomach to avoid nausea.** If we lack zinc; wounds take longer to heal; men may not notice the deficiency until they develop prostate problems. Zinc has 2.3 times better absorption as an amino acid chelate than as zinc sulfate. Typically, amino acid chelated zinc is retained twice as well as zinc fluoride. Important also is which amino-acids are used to form the chelate. Zinc and cadmium occur naturally in the earth. Zinc in the diet can prevent the assimilation of cadmium.
Zirconium	Zirconium is used to protect alloys from corrosion. Although it has no known biological role, the human body contains, on average, 250 mg of zirconium. It is used in medicine to offset hyperkalemia. High blood potassium levels are associated with cardiac arrhythmias, conduction system abnormalities, and increased mortality. In acute hyperkalemia. Zirconium cyclosilicate rapidly lowers potassium levels, thus delaying or potentially averting the need for emergent dialysis.

Table 8:   Well-researched Toxic Minerals (Metals)

Toxic Minerals (Metals)	
Name	Notes
Aluminum	Aluminum plays no biological role, but it is found in nature in large amounts. Aluminum hydroxide is used in some antacid preparations, but the aluminum is not converted into a product that can be eliminated from the system. We can pick up the level in a hair analysis. We also find aluminum in canned foods, foods wrapped in aluminum foil, in aluminum utensils, and in antiperspirants. These are the biggest sources, stay away from all of them. Once the aluminum is in the system, it can be removed using methionine, alginates, and a lot of vitamin C.
Arsenic	Arsenic is found in some skin lotions, hair dyes, medicines, water, seafood, some fruit, and in cigarette smoke. If found in the body, it is usually in the liver, bones, and hair. In cancer, there is an increased amount in the blood. Aside from the tars, arsenicals, etc. in cigarette smoke, the most important substance (which we are never told about) is sulfuric acid, used in the manufacture of the cigarette paper. Lung cancer is going up rapidly in females who smoke. One cigarette will destroy more vitamin C than you can eat in one day.
Cadmium	Zinc and cadmium occur naturally in the earth. Zinc in the diet can prevent the assimilation of cadmium. Too much cadmium is an important cause of anemia and emphysema; it also causes high blood pressure, arteriosclerosis, and heart disease. Poisoning results from ingestion of fumes. Other sources are: oyster, cigarettes, gasoline, rubber tires, heating oils, steelmaking, and lead and copper processing. We are putting six million pounds into our atmosphere each year.

Doctor to Patient

Toxic Minerals (Metals)	
Name	**Notes**
Lead	Lead and cadmium are toxic elements usually found in smokers. Sources of lead include toothpaste, hair dyes, airplane exhaust, alloys, asphalt, air conditioners, automobile exhaust, auto heaters, batteries, bone meal, building debris, ceramics, charcoal, coal-gas, cosmetics, dolomite, dust, dyes, fertilizers, gas burners, gasoline, leaded glass, hair shampoos, hair rinses, hair sprays, linotype, some milk, minerals, petroleum oils, paints, pencils, pesticides, pewter, plaster, poultry, print shops, printed paper, rain, road dust, rubber tires, scrap metals, smog, smoke, tobacco, forest fires, vegetables, water, water-pipes, welding, wine. Symptoms of lead poisoning include porphyria, kidney damage, a relationship to gout, memory loss, mental retardation, infertility, damage to the central nervous system, anemia, jaundice, liver malfunction, low blood levels of vitamin B6, vitamin C deficiency, pituitary damage, and reduced levels of blood proteins.
Mercury	Symptoms of mercury poisoning include pain in the left part of the chest, retinal bleeding, dim vision, film over eyes, dry eyes, grey ring around the cornea, red irritable throat, inflammation in the upper airways, pleurisy, difficulty in swallowing, severe amnesia, anxiety, irritability, difficulty to impossibility to control behavior, indecisiveness, loss of interest in life, tiredness, a feeling of being old, resistance to intellectual work, increased need for sleep, vertigo, headaches (often migraine type), facial paralysis, painful pull at the lower jaw toward the collar bone, increases salivation, a metallic taste (gallbladder), bleeding gums especially while bruising teeth, joint pain, lower back pain, muscle weakness, slow muscle action, pressure pains (needles) in the liver, asthmatic breathing, gastrointestinal irritation, eczema, needle-like sensations in lymph glands under the arm and in the groin.

Toxic Minerals (Metals)	
Name	Notes
Nickel	Nickel activates the enzymes arginase carboxylase and trypsin. It binds with protein to form nickeloplasmin, the function of which is not known. Nickel exposure causes formation of free radicals in various tissues in both human and animals which lead to various modifications to DNA bases, enhanced lipid peroxidation, and altered calcium and sulfhydryl homeostasis. Nickel inhibits acid phosphatase and is associated with cancer and some skin ailments. It is found in amalgam fillings, in stainless steel cooking utensils, as well as in some food and drinks, such as margarine and some decaffeinated coffees (not allowed in the Ellis program).

Table 9: Less Well-researched Toxic Minerals (Metals)

Other Toxic Metals	
Name	Notes
Antimony	Pure antimony is used in semiconductors, batteries, low friction metals, flame-proof materials, paints, ceramic enamels, glass, and pottery. Antimony is used as a medicine for parasitic infections, but exposure to relatively high concentrations of it can cause lung diseases, heart problems, diarrhea, severe vomiting, and stomach ulcers.
Barium	Barium is used in spark-plugs, vacuum tubes, and fluorescent lamps. It is used by the oil industry as drilling mud and by other manufacturers to make paint, tiles, glass, and rubber. Water-soluble barium compounds can be harmful to human health, causing paralyses and in some cases even death. Small amounts may cause breathing difficulties, elevated blood pressure, heart rhythm changes, stomach irritation, muscle weakness, changes in nerve reflexes, swelling of brains and liver, and kidney and heart damage.
Beryllium	Beryllium improves many physical properties when added as an alloying element to certain metals. It is used commonly in dental alloys. Approximately 35 micrograms of beryllium are found in the average human body, an amount not considered harmful. Beryllium is chemically similar to magnesium and therefore can displace it from enzymes, which causes them to malfunction.
Bismuth	Bismuth is the most naturally diamagnetic element, and has one of the lowest values of thermal conductivity among metals and is weakly radioactive. It is used in cosmetics, pigments, and a few pharmaceuticals, notably bismuth subsalicylate, used to treat diarrhea. Bismuth has unusually low toxicity for a heavy metal. As the toxicity of lead has become more apparent in recent years, there is an increasing use of bismuth alloys as a replacement for lead.

Other Toxic Metals	
Name	Notes
Platinum	Platinum is used to increase wear- and tarnish-resistance in fine jewelry. It and its alloys are used in surgical tools, laboratory utensils, wire, and electrical contact points. It is used in catalytic converters and in liquid crystal display glass. Platinum bonds are often applied as a medicine to cure cancer, but success is dependent upon the kind of bonds that are shaped and the exposure level and immunity of the patient. Although not a very dangerous metal, platinum salts can cause DNA damage, cancer, allergic reactions of the skin and the mucous membrane, damage to organs, such as intestines, kidneys and bone marrow, and a loss of hearing. It can also potentiate the toxicity of other dangerous chemicals in the body, such as selenium.
Silver	Silver is used in electrical contacts and conductors, specialized mirrors, catalysis of chemical reactions, and in photographic film and X-rays. Silver is also used in food coloring. Dilute silver nitrate solutions and other silver compounds are used as disinfectants and microbiocides (oligodynamic effect), added to bandages and wound-dressings, catheters and other medical instruments. Silver is used in water purifiers to prevent growth of bacteria and algae in filters. Silver plays no known natural biological role in humans and is not toxic to humans, but most silver salts are. In large doses, silver and compounds containing it can be absorbed into the circulatory system and become deposited in various body tissues, leading to argyria, which results in a blue-grayish pigmentation of the skin, eyes, and mucous membranes.

Nutritional Supplements

Other Toxic Metals	
Name	**Notes**
Strontium	Strontium burns in air, and because of its extreme reactivity with oxygen and water, this element occurs naturally only in compounds with other elements. It is kept under mineral oil or kerosene to prevent spontaneous ignition and oxidation. The primary use for strontium is in glass for color television cathode ray tubes to prevent X-ray emission. The human body absorbs strontium as if it were calcium. However, the stable forms of strontium do not pose a significant health threat. The radioactive form, Sr-90, can lead to various bone disorders and diseases, including bone cancer.
Thallium	Thallium is used in photoresistors and high-temperature superconducting materials for magnetic resonance imaging, storage of magnetic energy, magnetic propulsion, and electric power generation and transmission. Soluble thallium salts (many of which are nearly tasteless) are highly toxic and were used in rat poisons and insecticides. Thallium and its compounds are extremely toxic, and should be handled with great care. People can be exposed to thallium in the workplace by breathing it in, skin absorption, swallowing it, or eye contact. Contact with skin is dangerous, and adequate ventilation should be provided when melting this metal. Man-made sources of thallium pollution include gaseous emission of cement factories, coal burning power plants, and metal sewers. The main source of elevated thallium concentrations in water is the leaching of thallium from ore processing operations. Prussian Blue dye is used to rid the body of thallium.

Other Toxic Metals	
Name	Notes
Thorium	Thorium was commonly used as the light source in gas mantles, but this application has declined because of concerns about its radioactivity. Thorium is still widely used as an alloying element. It is also popular as a material in high-end optics and scientific instrumentation. The chemical toxicity of thorium is low because thorium and its most common compounds are poorly soluble in water. People who work with thorium compounds are at a risk of dermatitis. It can take as much as thirty years after the ingestion of thorium for symptoms to manifest themselves. Exposure to an aerosol of thorium, however, can lead to increased risk of cancers of the lung, pancreas, and blood, as lungs and other internal organs can be penetrated by alpha radiation. Exposure to thorium internally leads to increased risk of liver diseases.
Tin	About half of the tin produced is used in solder. The rest is divided among tin plating, tin chemicals, brass and bronze, and niche uses, such as production of PVC pipe and Lithium-ion batteries. Cases of poisoning from tin metal, its oxides, and its salts are almost nonexistent, but certain organotin compounds are almost as toxic as cyanide. People can be exposed to tin in the workplace by breathing it in, skin contact, and eye contact.
Titanium	Titanium is alloyed with iron, aluminium, vanadium, and molybdenum to produce strong, lightweight, non-corroding alloys. These are used in aerospace, military, manufacturing, desalination, and agri-food. Some products are medical prostheses, orthopedic implants, dental instruments, sporting goods, jewelry, and mobile phones. Titanium is non-toxic even in large doses and does not play any natural role inside the human body. It does, however, sometimes accumulate in tissues that contain silica.

Other Toxic Metals	
Name	**Notes**
Uranium	Originally, uranium was used in glass making and in photographic chemicals. Now, the major application of uranium in the military sector is in high-density penetrators. Depleted uranium is also used as a shielding material in some containers used to store and transport radioactive materials. Uranium-235 has been used as the explosive material to produce nuclear weapons. The main use of uranium in the civilian sector is to fuel nuclear power plants. A person can be exposed to uranium by inhaling dust in air or by ingesting contaminated water and food. Most ingested uranium is excreted during digestion. After entering the bloodstream, the absorbed uranium tends to bioaccumulate and stay for many years in bone tissue because of uranium's affinity for phosphates. Normal functioning of the kidney, brain, liver, heart, and other systems can be affected by uranium exposure, because, besides being weakly radioactive, uranium is a toxic metal.

Emulsified Vitamins and Coenzymes

When you ingest the oil-soluble vitamin A suspended in an emulsion, instead of it being picked up in the portal system, it is picked up in the lymphatic system. When the lymphatics pick it up, it goes up through the cisterna chyli and empties into the inferior vena cava just before it goes into the heart. It's in the bloodstream and goes directly to the affected cell, and the cell picks it out of the bloodstream before it ever goes through on its second pass into the portal system. Then, much of the vitamin is destroyed in the liver. The cells have the first opportunity to get it.

What we're trying to do is use emulsions of oil and water. We use sesame oil in making these emulsions, and can put vitamin A and vitamin E together if we choose. **Conventional vitamin A supplements must be taken carefully.** Many references tell you to take 100,000 units of vitamin A. However, if you were to take that much vitamin A in the little gel capsules on a daily basis for 30 to 60 days, it could kill you.

In the therapy of Dr. Hans Nieper of Germany, nine million units of emulsified vitamin A have been given on a daily basis with only slight toxic effects. In cancer work, they use three million units on a daily basis. I take somewhere around 750,000 units of vitamin A every day in the emulsion form with no harmful effects. I have been on this for over a year. We're doing the same thing with emulsified vitamin E that is 300% more potent than any other form of vitamin E.

Digestive Aids

Although the main function of digestion is to convert the foods that we eat into energy, the digestive system has even more functions. It is the main area of contact with an external environment full of bacteria, protozoa, fungi, viruses, and many toxic substances. To deal with these insults, the digestive tract is infiltrated with a large number of immune cells in what is called gut-associated lymphoid tissue (GALT). This is a very important part of mucosal-associated lymphoid tissue (MALT) representing almost 70% of the entire immune system. Approximately 80% of plasma cells reside in GALT, standing by to issue an immune response to whatever antigens appear in the tract.

If your digestive system were working at top efficiency, you would feel good after eating, you would have no symptoms of indigestion, and your next bowel movement would be well-formed and without discomfort. To understand an ideal digestive process and to indicate stages when and what digestive aids might be necessary, refer to Table 10.

Table 10: Ideal Digestion vs. Need for Digestive Aids

Stage	Place	Ideal Outcome (Simplified)	Difficulty	Digestive Aid/Action
Mastication	Mouth	Food is converted from solid to small-particle, liquid form by extensive chewing.	Inability to chew properly, either through lack of teeth or paralysis.	None, except for blending food before consumption. Even blended material should be given an opportunity to mix with saliva.
Alkaline Hydrolysis	Mouth	Food particles are thoroughly mixed with the alkaline enzyme ptyalin (alpha-amylase) to digest starches (carbohydrates) and trigger the digestive process. Starches should be digested as completely as possible down to short-chain saccharides during this stage.	Inability to produce sufficient saliva. Undigested carbohydrates ferment and interfere with acidic environment in the stomach.	None. Although the amylase enzyme is found in enzyme supplements, taking them by mouth serves no purpose in the mouth. Liquid phosphorus as a digestive aid is beneficial to phosphorylate sugars at the initial steps of energy metabolism.

Stage	Place	Ideal Outcome (Simplified)	Difficulty	Digestive Aid/Action
Acid Hydrolysis	Stomach	The alkaline bolus coming from the mouth through the pharynx and esophagus and into the stomach triggers the production of strongly acidic stomach secretions essential to the breakdown of proteins.	Inability to produce sufficient hydrochloric acid in the stomach causes protein to linger in the stomach and be subject to putrefaction.	Betaine hydrochloride tablets or apple cider vinegar taken approximately one hour after the meal to allow stomach to produce as much natural secretions as possible.

Nutritional Supplements

Stage	Place	Ideal Outcome (Simplified)	Difficulty	Digestive Aid/Action
Fat Digestion and Absorption of Various Digested Materials	Small Intestine	The acidic bolus coming from the stomach passes through the pyloric valve into the duodenum of the small intestine. There it is exposed to bile that neutralizes the acid and pancreatic enzymes that digest fats, as well as carbohydrates and protein.	(1) Insufficient hydrochloric acid in the stomach cannot overcome highly alkaline bile leaking back into the stomach through the pyloric valve, causing an alkaline "heartburn." (2) Individuals without gallbladders may not have have sufficient bile secretions after a meal.	(1) Betaine hydrochloride tablets or apple cider vinegar taken at the onset of discomfort may relieve the indigestion and bitter taste in the mouth. (2) Given that hydrochloric acid secretion is complete, bile salts in tablet form may be necessary to continue the digestive process at this stage.

Stage	Place	Ideal Outcome (Simplified)	Difficulty	Digestive Aid/Action
Nutrient Absorption	Large Intestine	Digested materials to be absorbed, such as amino acids and simple sugars, are picked up by the capillaries of the large intestine and pass through the portal vein into the liver and on to the bloodstream. Fatty acids are taken into the lymph system through the thoracic duct and carried to the bloodstream. Water and salts are also absorbed. Appropriate bacteria act on the bolus, producing beneficial substances such as vitamins.	Disturbance of the intestinal environment can occur from improper diet, alcohol consumption, and smoking. The population of bacteria may not be optimal, allowing fermentation of carbohydrates, putrefaction of proteins, and rancidification of fats. Diarrhea or constipation may result.	The long-term solution is a program of cleansing the intestines, no more frequent than a monthly basis, treating inflammation with raw cabbage juice and/or aloe vera gel before bedtime, and repopulating the intestine with beneficial bacteria by taking high potency lactobacillus capsules (probiotics) after each cleansing.

Glandulars (Protomorphogens)

Glandulars, or protomorphogens, as Dr. Royal Lee called them, are nutritional supplements made from organs and tissues of cattle. Use of such materials is not new, as they have been used by health practitioners for over 100 years. Originally, protomorphogens were available as injectables, which were very effective, but the drug companies pressured the FDA to ban this form in the United States. Proponents of glandular therapy were forced to find another way to deliver them to the body, so they developed ingestible forms.

The basis for glandular therapy is that degeneration of an organ can be offset or reversed through ingestion of the tissue of that particular organ. Degeneration occurs when the cells of the organ are damaged and debris from the cells are released into the bloodstream. The body makes antibodies to the debris that can also attack the original organ. This is a manifestation of autoimmune disease, such as diabetes, rheumatoid arthritis, and neuromuscular disorders.

Do Protomorphogens Work?

One of the criticisms I have heard is that protomorphogens taken by mouth must be completely broken by digestive enzymes into fats, carbohydrates, and amino acids. Therefore, there would be no significant, biologically-active fragments, such as enzymes, hormones, and DNA sequences to be assimilated in the whole. To counter this notion, I recommend Dr. Royal Lee's and Bill Hansen's book, *Protomorphology*. It is a toughie and you need to be a good biochemist to understand it.

These protomorphogens work; we see them working all of the time. Most criticism comes from doctors and Ph.D.s who have no clinical practice and are just theoretical chemists. But remember, minerals make the enzyme systems, and vitamins are the catalysts that make the minerals and protein become the enzymes. There are certain minerals that will work with the protomorphogens, but again, total balancing is what we want.

Most of the time we give them to you with meals. Like Standard Process' Cardiotrophin, the protomorphogen for the heart, is given one tablet three times a day (t.i.d.). If you have a lot of spasm we'll give you their Cardio Plus that contains a lot of vitamin E2. It is an antispasmodic. People with a lot of angina pain take nitroglycerin, but if they take vitamin E2, it'll do a better job and relieve the pain. Also nitroglycerin has to be broken down in the liver, and it breaks your liver down. You protect the patient by getting them off nitroglycerine and putting them on vitamin E2. It also has vitamin B2 in it.

Adjunct Supplements

An adjunct supplement is usually considered as a non-essential substance or compound added to the diet to perform a particular function or variety of functions. It is usually not taken for a single pharmacological effect. The following are examples of adjunct supplements.

Aloe Vera

Aloe vera has been used both as an anti-inflammatory to treat mildly inflamed mucous membranes of the mouth, throat, and digestive tract. It has also been shown to relieve diabetic neuropathy.

Bioflavonoids

Bioflavonoids (biologically active flavonoids) are found in plants, fruits and vegetables and are consumed by animals and humans. Bioflavonoids are beneficial in improving connective tissue, local circulation, and the collagen matrix; and in protection of collagen against non-enzymatic proteolytic activity. They are also protective against alveolar bone loss in periodontal disease. As free radical scavengers, flavonoids inhibit lipid peroxidation, promote vascular relaxation, and help prevent atherosclerosis.

Carnitine

Carnitine is found mainly in animal tissues. Lysine and methionine are needed to make L-carnitine, but the useful form is produced only in the liver, brain, and kidneys. Muscles take up carnitine from the bloodstream and contain most of the body's carnitine stores. L-carnitine transfers fatty acids to the mitochondria where they undergo oxidation to regenerate coenzyme A, a vital part of energy metabolism. Defective L-carnitine metabolism has been shown in individuals with diabetes mellitus, malignancies, myocardial ischemia, and alcohol abuse.

Editor: More information about carnitine can be found at the WebMD webpage: http://www.webmd.com/vitamins-supplements/ ingredientmono-1026-l-carnitine.aspx?activeingredientid=1026.

Co-Enzyme Q10 (CoQ10)

CoQ10 is an important cofactor in the transfer of electrons in energy metabolism. It is an effective antioxidant that participates in the function of cellular membranes and stimulates the growth of new cells.

Fish Oils

Omega-3 polyunsaturated fatty acids are found in fish oils, such as those from cod, salmon, tuna, and halibut. It is also found in krill, plants, algae, and nuts. Omega-3 fatty acids are important to brain function and in normal growth and development.

When the oil is taken by itself, the liver, which acts like a sponge, removing vitamins A and D-3 before they can be distributed throughout the body. However, when emulsified oil is taken on an empty stomach, it goes directly into the bloodstream, passing easily to places where the active vitamins are needed.

Superoxide Dismutase (SOD)

Superoxide Dismutase is an enzyme associated with copper, zinc, manganese, and iron. It catalyzes the dismutation reaction of toxic superoxides (free radicals) to molecular oxygen and hydrogen peroxide. Three forms of superoxide dismutase are present in humans. SOD1 is located in the cytoplasm, SOD2 in the mitochondria, and SOD3 is extracellular. SOD1 and SOD3 contain copper and zinc, whereas SOD2, the mitochondrial enzyme, has manganese in its reactive centre. Manganese and zinc stimulate production of SOD.

Herbs

Herbs are plants used as flavorings and spices in cooking, but herbs can also be used as supplements for health or medicinal reasons. They are also referred to as botanicals, which are substances obtained from plants and used in food supplements, personal care products, or pharmaceuticals. Other names include herbal medicine and plant medicine.

There are many brands of herbs available, and I am not well-schooled in their use. One must be careful; some herbs can interact with certain medications, including those for high blood pressure, diabetes, and depression, as well as blood thinners and even over-the-counter drugs. **Also, do not take too many herb capsules. More is not necessarily better, and it could be dangerous. My concern is overuse of herb concoctions and the possibility of their causing regional inflammations in the digestive tract.** Therefore, consult a competent herbalist.

Editor: The website of Dr. John Christopher is http://www.drchristopher.com/.

A Word About Homeopathy

Homeopathy is defined as the treatment of a disease by small doses of natural substances that, in a healthy person, produces symptoms of that particular disease. However, I believe that homeopathy is the use of any vitamin, mineral, or drug in small amounts. For example, instead of using 300,000 units of penicillin, which is a typical dose, use only 1/6 or 1/12 millionth of a unit.

Homeopathy has proven to me that you can use very small amounts if you know how to put supplements into the system on a proper basis. Homeopathy does a very wonderful job as an activator to what you have in your body. The goal is for the penicillin to act only as a catalyst to help the body do its own job. We are finding that a lot of the protomorphogens that we use are better in smaller dosages. In fact, if a value in the bloodwork is not too far off from desired, we may use only one protomorphogen per day. Most of the time, we use three.

Nutritional Supplements

8   Feet and Posture

Start with the feet, or you are defeated before you start!

I begin this chapter with one of my favorite sayings to emphasize the importance of the feet to the health of the entire body. Did you ever stop to think how important your feet are? First, you should realize that 1/4 of all of the bones of the body are located in just the two feet — 26 bones in each one! The feet represent the foundation of the bony structure of the entire body; **it is of tremendous importance that the bones be balanced properly, otherwise any discrepancy, even in one foot, creates a short leg and a resultant spinal curvature.** As a result, the vitality of the body is lowered at least 10%, based on my own research during which I treated the feet of over 100,000 persons.

Modern Shoe Construction

The shoes made today, regardless of the quality of the leather, are not constructed properly. To save money, the manufacturers have neglected to include a substantial steel shank — the part that joins and supports the shoe from midfront to heel. A strong shank is absolutely necessary to prevent the anterior portion of the calcaneus (os calcis or heel bone) from rotating downward, with concomitant internal rotation of the cuboid bone. This movement causes a depressed fourth metatarsal and an elevated fifth metatarsal.

The visual indicator of improper shoes is the relative positioning of the toes. Let the feet dangle down and look at the alignment of the toes, all of which should lie on the same plane. If they do not, the bones in the foot are out of position and need to be corrected.

Misalignment of the toes indicates that the middle of the shoe is flexing downward toward the floor with every step. The sole probably makes a quiet slapping sound. There is little or no support between the heel and the sole, and the foot becomes fatigued and painful. To treat this condition, the foot should be manipulated and the calcaneus supported by a felt pad affixed to the insole; further, wedge-soled or well-shanked shoes should be worn. Women have a more difficult time finding properly-constructed dress shoes. To acquaint yourself with possible conditions that can be caused by incorrectly-supported shoes, see Figure 3, below.

5 VITAL POINTS

Five vital points of the body that may be affected with incorrect shoe support.

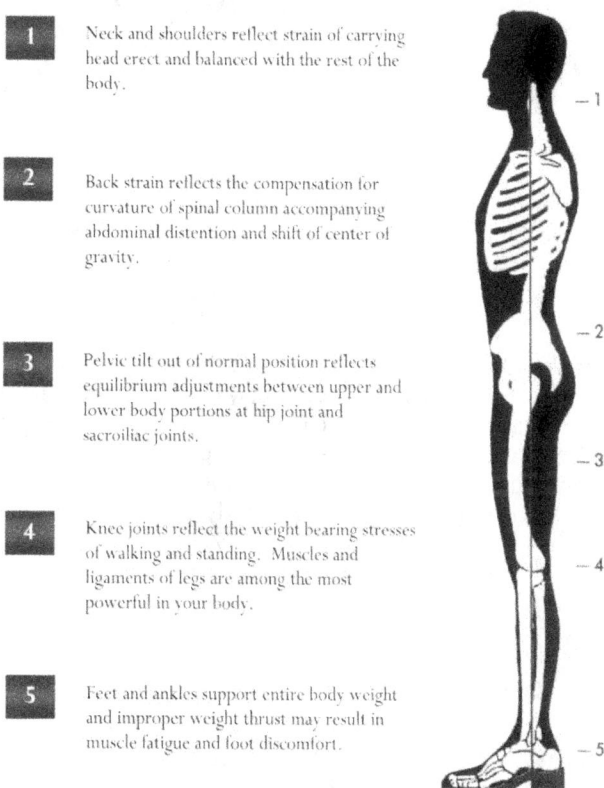

1 Neck and shoulders reflect strain of carrying head erect and balanced with the rest of the body.

2 Back strain reflects the compensation for curvature of spinal column accompanying abdominal distention and shift of center of gravity.

3 Pelvic tilt out of normal position reflects equilibrium adjustments between upper and lower body portions at hip joint and sacroiliac joints.

4 Knee joints reflect the weight bearing stresses of walking and standing. Muscles and ligaments of legs are among the most powerful in your body.

5 Feet and ankles support entire body weight and improper weight thrust may result in muscle fatigue and foot discomfort.

Figure 3: Five vital points chart, used by permission, Foot-So-Port Shoe Corporation.

Functions of the Feet

Let's understand something about proper functioning of the feet.

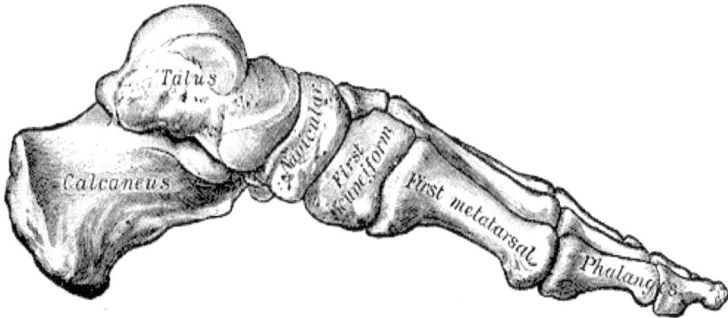

Figure 4:   Left foot medial view. From *Gray's Anatomy*, 1918.

First, we should consider the os calcis, or calcaneus, better known as the heelbone. To find out if you are standing correctly, have someone look at your foot and lower leg from the back as you stand on a hard surface. If the inner side of the Achilles tendon is perfectly straight, perpendicular to the floor, this is the normal position.

The more that the Achilles tendon bows to the inside (the medial side), the weaker the foot. Contrary to what you may have been told, flat feet are the strongest feet; the higher the arch, the weaker the foot. The heelbone is the rudder of the foot. If not held in the proper position, it may rotate inward, creating a pronation, or it may drop, but this motion depends on the relative orientation of the bone directly in front of the heelbone, the cuboid.

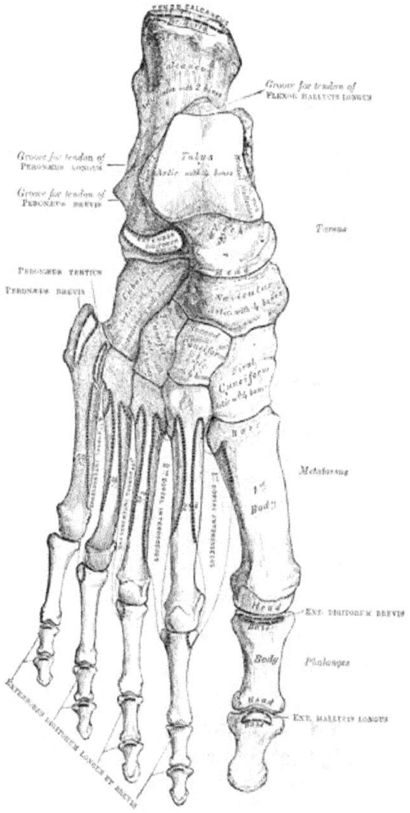

Figure 5: The right foot shown from the dorsal surface.
From *Gray's Anatomy*, 1918.

I consider the cuboid to be the most important bone of the foot. This bone, at its posterior/superior aspect has a twist facet under the os calcis to hold it in its position. The cuboid can rotate inward and downward, thus allowing the os calcis to either pronate or drop straight forward down in front. This problem can be easily seen in the walking pattern. The cuboid controls the fourth and the fifth metatarsal.

Other bones that play major roles in foot function are the navicular, or pivotal, bone; the talus; and the three cuneiforms, each of which controls a metatarsal bone. The interior cuneiform controls the motion of the first metatarsal, the middle cuneiform controls the motion of the second metatarsal, and the external cuneiform controls the motion of the third metatarsal.

Walking Patterns

In a normal walking gait, 60% of the body's weight is carried on the heel. As the weight is transferred to the toes, the load is distributed along the outer side of the foot, along the styloid process, then to the fifth toe, then to the fourth, as the foot rolls to the inside, the fifth metatarsal carries approximately 30% of the weight. Then the load is transferred to the big toe, which carries 10% of the weight. The big toe produces the greatest part of the push during forward propulsion. **If the feet slap, lacking a smooth transition of the weight from the heel to the ball of the foot, the cuboid has probably rotated inward and downward.**

Shoe Construction and Fit

Shoes are man-made contraptions. God made us to go barefoot, but with today's concrete, wood, and asphalt surfaces, there is too much potential for shock to allow it. **The rule in selecting a pair of shoes is to stay as close to nature as possible to accommodate the dimension and uninhibited motion of the foot. Don't fit your eyes; fit your feet! Think first of normal function and forget style.**

Bunions

If shoes are too pointed, too narrow, or too short, they can cause bunions (a dislocated big toe) and talar bunions (a dislocated little toe). The worst bunion I have ever seen involved the big toe being dislocated so far as to be over or under the other toes! In such a case, the best treatment would be surgery. However, the best preventive measure is wearing hose of the proper length and well-fitted shoes with low heels. It is very important that the toes be allowed freedom of motion within the shoe.

Anyone who has bunions should do the following one to three times every day. Expect the full effect not to take place for one to two years of daily application.

1. Grasp the foot, holding the first metatarsal with the base of the thumb and first finger.
2. With the other hand, grasp the big toe (or the little toe in case of a talar bunion).

3. Pull the toe away from the foot and rotate it in both directions for several minutes. This exercise does cause some discomfort because it makes the muscles and ligaments go back to work, whereas they had been relaxed. Try not to cause too much pain or inflammation.

Vericose Veins

Rotation of the cuboid is common today, because modern shoes are manufactured with flat or concave arches and without a steel shank. These deficiencies in design allow the cuboid bone to rotate inward and downward. The styloid process is out and up; the fourth toe is down; and the fifth toe is up. This is evidence that the cuboid has rotated. As this bone is also attached to muscles that run around the foot to the outside, a tightening of the musculature of the lower leg is usually experienced. This tightening leads to the development of varicose veins in the legs of many persons. It also causes the tibia and fibula to rotate, constricting the interossus membrane, which narrows the space needed for the veins of the calf to work properly. Blood is forced into the smaller external veins, producing vericosities.

Callouses

If one develops a callous on the bottom of the foot, the usual cause is the inward rotation of the cuboid, thereby flattening the cuneiforms and allowing the metatarsals to drop. The excessive amount of pressure and friction that is put on the metatarsal arch causes the callous. A callous is nature's way of protecting the tender, sensitive areas underneath the skin. The excessive amount of pressure can cause a plantar wart, a very difficult problem. Restoration of the proper relationship of the cuboid to the other bones of the foot is aided by the use of the cuboid pad. This pad is 1/8" thick, 1 1/4" wide, and from 1 1/2" to 3" long, depending on the size of the shoe. The pad should be 1/4" to 1/2" behind the heads of the metatarsals and never directly under them and extend to just in front of the calcaneus.

Socks and Hose

Serious problems result from the wearing of short hose. The way to test hose is to stand in your stocking feet and look at them. Unless you have excess hose extending past your toes, you are wearing them too short. Women have the greatest problem with hose, because they must wear them wrinkle-free, therefore too tight! The pulling back on the toes produces bunions and talar bunions. Short hose cause hammer toes, a condition in which the toes are flexed. The tendons tighten and hold the toes in that position so that they cannot effectively balance the body as they are called upon to carry their part of the load in walking.

Heel Height

Men should never wear a heel height exceeding 1"! A man's pelvis allows him to withstand only 1" elevation of the heel relative to the level of the ball of the foot. This revelation excludes many of the boot types, especially cowboy boots. That style of boot was developed for the purpose of keeping the foot in the stirrup — not for walking!

Men in cowboy boots and women in high heels have more severe problems with heel height. The first thing to remember is that, for every forward movement, you have a backward movement. Right? So when you get on those high heels, you raise your heels up in the air. That means one thing — you have a backward movement in the ankles. To offset that, you have to have a forward movement, so your knees go forward. Because your knees go forward, you have to have one that goes backward so your rump goes backward. When your rump goes backward, you have to have a counter movement forward, so your shoulders go forward. When your shoulders go forward, your head goes up in the air!

In my work as educational and research director for an orthopedic shoe company, I had the opportunity to participate in many different studies. In one, we varied the heel heights of womens' shoes and used X-ray photography to record the influence of these changes on the feet, ankles, knees, and pelvises. The heels were varied from 1/4" to 2" in 1/4" increments; above that, they were varied in 1" increments to 3", 4", 5", and 6". Pictures were taken of each woman's feet without shoes and with shoes of each of the heel heights. We found that the womens' pelvises can withstand up to, but not over, a heel higher than a 1 1/2" heel — what is called in the shoe business a "12-8 heel." For every 1/8" that the heel is raised above the 1 1/2" height, the pelvis is tipped forward seven degrees, and it locks. The uterus keeps going backward and ends up on the rectum, as a retroverted uterus. The locking is a result of the fifth lumbar vertrebra going so far forward that it could not regain normal motion.

If ladies are having problems with their backs or menstrual cycles, the heels on their shoes are most likely too high. Ladies wearing three-, four-, and five-inch heels will wind up with menstrual problems, most likely ending with a hysterectomy. The twisting effect also interferes with the functioning of the ovaries in producing estrogen and progesterone and throwing the cycle out of balance. Women should not wear a heel height over 1 1/2" if they want good posture, more vitality, and mental acuity.

Exercise for Weak Feet

Whenever there is a weakness, there is inward rotation of the os calcis, a condition called pronation. The more that the Achilles tendon slants toward the inner side of the foot, the more severe the weakness. This condition can be alleviated by the comprehensive exercise described below.

Before you fall asleep at night or before you get out of bed in the morning, do the following:

1. Extend both feet off the end of the bed, placing the Achilles tendon even with the edge of the mattress.

2. Flex (curl) the toes down as far as possible. Keep the toes in this position during the entire exercise.

3. Bend both feet upward, toward the shins, keeping the toes curled.

4. Bend both feet downward, away from the shins, keeping the toes curled.

5. Alternate these two movements, counting an up/down movement of both as one repetition. Do 100 repetitions. This movement exercises the arch. Anticipate that you cannot do more than 20 repetitions without the muscles beginning to cramp.

6. When a cramp develops, stop and rest.

7. Continue until the goal of 100 is reached.

When you can do 100 repetitions without cramping, you will probably discover that your feet are functioning perfectly.

Strapping the Feet and Ankles

Athletes should properly strap their feet before competition. The objective is to create pressure against the internal cuneiform, the cuboid, and the styloid process of the fifth metatarsal bone as one is walking, jogging, or running. This pressure creates an upward force to the middle and external cuneiforms and the inner aspects of the cuboid. 60% of the blood comes down the leg, under the sustentaculum tali bone (juts out) on the inner side of the ankle, and into the plantar arch blood vessels. 40% of the blood goes into the front part of the foot. The tape creates a pump action as it pushes the arch up when the foot contacts the ground and releases the arch when the foot is recovering before making contact with the ground again. An increase in circulation is afforded the entire foot and, as a result, the feet do not become tired.

Over the years, including my own stint in professional basketball, I have wrapped the feet of my own teammates after manipulation while a game was in progress! For example, using these techniques of strapping after a first half let the player participate in the second half without any further problems or complications.

Strapping the feet also helps to prevent sprained ankles. Sprained ankles involve three foot bones that are prone to becoming jammed (limitation of motion) during normal use. The most important one is the cuboid, which rotates inward and downward. The middle cuneiform is a triangular bone that becomes a wedge. As the foot spreads, the middle cuneiform lowers to a point between the internal and external cuneiforms and locks the two in place. The third jam occurs where the tibia inserts forward of the talus.

To check this relationship, try to put your finger in a depression, or hollow spot, on the top of the talus. If the tibia has moved too far forward, you cannot get your finger into the depression. In some cases the tibia goes into a stuck position. The position of the displaced bones causes the slapping of the foot during walking, and the ankle is not given its desired range of motion. The foot plainly cannot operate properly!

Those of us who believe in the benefits of manipulation are far superior in helping patients with sprained ankles than those who are not inclined to use manipulative techniques. These three bones must be put back into their proper relationship so that they can move normally. If they are never put back, one will have a chronic foot and/or ankle problem for the rest of his or her life.

Foot Strapping Method

To strap the feet, use non-waterproof adhesive tape. Application is rather simple and can be done by the performer without the aid of a trainer or doctor. Use two strips of non-allergenic, non-waterproof adhesive tape that are 1 1/2" wide and of sufficient length to encircle the foot and overlap on the dorsal surface (instep). Follow these directions:

1. Place the first strip on the bottom surface of the foot so that the front edge of the tape is slightly in front of the head of the fifth metatarsal. Make sure that there are no wrinkles in the tape.

2. Bring the tape up on the outside, over the instep, pulling it taut (not tight; do not stretch the skin). The only tape that is put on tight is that which directly contacts the sole.

3. Bring up the tape on the inside, overlapping the tape from the outside and pulling it taut, as well. Relax the tape and let it literally fall over itself, following the contour of the foot and overlapping itself.

4. Place the second strip overlapping the first strip by 1/8" uniformly all the way around. Apply it in the same way as the first strip. These two strips should cover the posterior transverse arch and the posterior metatarsal arch.

5. After competition, remove the tape by loosening the end of the tape that was last applied and drawing it back over itself in the direction that it was applied.

Ankle Strapping Method

This method is used to keep the foot in the proper lateral position by preventing the foot from inverting and everting, while allowing the foot to flex and extend normally. The limitation of lateral motion prevents the sprain from taking place. Replace the tape every 24 hours to avoid irritation and possible blistering. Use two strips of non-allergenic, non-waterproof adhesive tape 2" wide and approximately 28" long. Follow these directions:

1. Apply the tape approximately 12" vertically, up the outside of the leg.

2. Turn (evert) the foot to the outside and pull the tape underneath the foot and around to the inner side. Press the tape, making sure that there are no wrinkles on the bottom.

3. When you have the foot in that position, turn the entire foot to the inside (invert) as far as it will go.

4. Pull the tape around, letting it wrap around and adhere to the leg in an easy manner. Let it fall into place and adhere to the inner side of the leg vertically, until it reaches approximately 12" above the ankle.

5. Place the second strip of tape vertically, across the forward part of the tibia, overlapping the first tape.

6. Turn the foot to the outside (evert), pull the tape taut on the outside, and apply it to the bottom of the foot. Press the tape, making sure that there are no wrinkles on the bottom.

7. Turn the fore part of the foot to the inside (invert) and let the tape run up vertically and adhere to the leg as before.

Additional tape may be applied over these strips for additional support.

Anatomical Short Leg - A Major Problem

In the late 1930s, I was part of a study of children of the Three Rivers, Michigan school system. Further, I was involved in a similar study of mentally deficient children in a special school in St. Louis, Missouri. The children of grades 1, 3, 5, 7, 9, 11, and 12 were checked on three consecutive years with a posture check machine, while the teachers kept track of the IQ scores. **These studies revealed that 62% of all of the students we checked had an anatomical short leg, meaning that one leg was at least 1/8" shorter than the other.** Corrections of these deficiencies raised the IQ scores an average of 10%. Uncorrected deficients tended to have more irritations in the feet, legs, and spine than those with legs of equal lengths. As recent as 1980, researchers at the Michigan State Osteopathic College reported that 60% of the persons that they checked had an anatomical short leg. **Of course, we are talking about a true, structurally short leg, based on the length of the bones and not on any muscular tension that may give the impression of a short leg.**

The lumbar vertebrae will rotate in a direction toward the anatomical short leg. However, if there has been some type of accident that has twisted the spine, the rotation may be in the opposite direction. This is why it is necessary to take a standing postural X-ray in an anterior-posterior plane, as well as in a lateral plane. It may be advisable to use a larger plate so that the plate extends approximately 2" below the acetabulum.

Our own research, described above, revealed that the greatest irritation was caused by a difference in leg length of 1/8" to 3/16". Differences in this range cause an imbalance at the base of the sacrum, creating a twist in the entire pelvic girdle. I have a 1/4" buildup on my right side because my right leg is a 1/4" shorter than my left. As long as I wear this, I don't have any back pain. If don't put it on my shoe, I use 10 times more energy every day than I should be using. It is very vital that you find somebody that can do this type of X-ray work.

To correct the rotation, it is necessary to add a lift, or shim, under both the sole and heel of the anatomical short leg. Unfortunately, over the years, we have heard so many so-called authorities — even some of my colleagues — state that all one needs is a heel lift. Nothing could be further from the truth. If we raise the heel without raising the sole, the spine is thrown into a torsion that is worse than would happen if no lift had been added at all! Therefore it is imperative that both the sole and heel be lifted by the same amount.

Feet and Posture

9 Common Health Issues

Editor: This chapter contains remarks made by Dr. Ellis about various health issues and how he preferred to address certain conditions. **No opinion contained herein, regardless of how thoughtful it seems, constitutes a complete method of treating a particular disease or condition.** Dr. Ellis emphasized that no one should expect nutritional modalities to act like drugs in giving immediate relief for a condition or render a decisive pharmacological effect. **It is imperative that anyone with a serious disorder seek a thorough evaluation by a trusted medical professional and follow sound medical advice resulting from the evaluation.**

This chapter contains thoughts on several common health issues, their significance, and what may be done to offset them.

"Acid Indigestion"

See Ulcers on page 189.

Aluminum Toxicity

Aluminum hydroxide is used in some antacid preparations, antiperspirants, and in baking powder, but the aluminum is not converted into a product that can be eliminated from the system. We can pick up the level in a hair analysis. We also find aluminum in canned foods, foods wrapped in aluminum foil, and in aluminum utensils. These are the biggest sources, stay away from all of them.

Antiperspirants that contain aluminum block the third passage of elimination of poisons out of your body. If you've got body odor, it's because your bowel is not working properly and it's kicking the poison out of your pores. If you have bad breath (the fourth passage of elimination), most of it comes from the undigested food in your stomach. You can get breath odor from periodontal diseases and gums, but it's minor compared to the amount caused by the gut. Once the aluminum is in the system, it can be removed using methionine, alginates, and a lot of vitamin C.

Arthritis

Arthritis occurs when the body attempts to maintain a proper level of blood serum albumin, the protein that normally covers joint surfaces. when the albumin level drops, protein is pulled into the bloodstream from the joint. The calcium that is left behind lays down a rough surface on the bone, and it becomes irritated during movement. If the albumin loss continues, a chronic painful arthritic condition results. **Cortisone relieves arthritis because it makes the body draw albumin from the muscles to raise the bloodstream concentration and to serve the joints. The joints, so supplied, show a decrease in irritability and inflammation until cortisone's effect wears off and the supply of looted protein from the muscles is cut off.** The first step in stopping protein thievery is to have ample, assimilable protein in the diet. Digestion of protein must be efficient and complete. Supplement with calcium, magnesium, manganese, phosphorus, and protein.

One of the good things for the pain of arthritis is to take a potato, cut it in half, take a teaspoon and scrape it and eat the scrapings. It'll take your pain out of an arthritis. But if you cut a piece out and eat the potato, it does not work; you must scrape it with a teaspoon.

Arthritis (Reactive)

Reactive arthritis was once called Reiter's Disease. See the Editor's note under Osteoporosis.

Back Pain (Lower Back/Anatomical Short Leg)

Low back pain is one of the most common complaints that a practitioner hears. It may originate from a number of causes, with a multiplicity of associated symptoms.

Causes

I can safely say that the majority of patients with low back pain have had other conditions associated with the primary complaint. These include:

- **Physical stress on the spine** with muscular imbalances and postural defects resulting from an anatomical short leg. See Feet and Posture on page 149.
- **Irritation of the internal organs and tissues** served by the nerves emanating from the lumbar and surrounding areas. Such irritation is commonly initiated by a toxic bowel. Avoid alkaline-forming foods (raise urine pH) in favor of acid-forming ones. See Detoxification on page 97.
- **Protein insufficiency,** with resultant hypothyroidism, immune deficiency, lack of muscular tone, and inefficient mineral transport through the bloodstream. See Protein Intake on page 46.
- **Mineral imbalances** brought about by inattention to proper dietary habits and vicarious patterns of supplementation. See Food and Diet on page 53 and Nutritional Supplements on page 113.
- **Inflammation and infection** of the prostate, uterus, bladder, etc., with accompanying alkalinity of the body fluids and regional hypoxia (poor oxygenation) within the affected tissues. See Acid-Alkaline Balance on page 49

Anatomical Short Leg

Studies show that 60-62% of the population has an anatomical short leg, meaning that one leg is at least 1/8" shorter than the other. Uncorrected deficients tend to have more irritations in the feet, legs, and spine than those with legs of equal lengths. Two conditions commonly encountered are generalized lower back pain and sciatica.

The one and only way to determine an anatomical short leg is in a standing position, as follows.

1. Take your clothes off and stand in front of a full-length mirror. If a hip is high on one side, a shoulder is high on one side, or if one breast is lower on one side, you've got a curvature in the spine that probably is caused by an anatomical short leg. Sixty-two percent of the hundreds of persons we tested in the 1930s had an anatomical short leg.

2. Put your thumbs on the crest of your ilia (outermost part of your hips) in exactly the same place on both sides, making sure that your feet are even with each other and squared to the mirror. If your legs are the same length, a line drawn between your thumbs should be perfectly level. The difference in the distance between your thumbs

and the floor are indicators of the difference in the length of your legs.

A postural doctor, especially a good osteopath or chiropractor, will do a standing X-ray front to back through an anterior/posterior lateral from the side of the lumbar, spine, and pelvis. Then he or she can measure the base of the sacrum to see how much it takes to get it back into a horizontal plane. That represents the thickness of the lift you apply to the sole and heel of the shoe on the short side.

What do you need to do about it? **To correct the rotation, it is necessary to add a lift, or shim, under both the sole and heel of the anatomical short leg.** Unfortunately, over the years, we have heard so many so-called authorities — even some of my colleagues — state that all one needs is a heel lift. Nothing could be further from the truth. If we raise the heel without raising the sole, the spine is thrown into a torsion that is worse than would happen if no lift had been added at all! **Therefore it is imperative that both the sole and heel be lifted by the same amount.** I estimate that persons with uncorrected anatomical short legs use 10 times the energy to accomplish the same tasks as if the problem were corrected.

Do not be fooled if a doctor checks your leg length while you are lying on a table, manipulates you, and claims to have corrected the short leg. He is not only fooling you; he is fooling himself! It is not possible to correct the length of leg bones through adjustment of the spine.

Blood Pressure Elevation

The common treatment for elevated, or high, blood pressure usually involves the long term use of diuretics. The first thing diuretics do is eliminate potassium from the system. You see, sodium is high on the inside of a blood vessel, potassium is high on the outside of a blood vessel. Nerves are just the opposite. Potassium is high on the inside of the nerve; sodium is high on the outside of the nerve. In the bloodwork, we use a ratio of sodium to potassium (Na/P) between 28/1 and 30/1. A ratio above or below that range means that you have broken down the nerve centers of the body. So it is vitally important that we understand what we are doing with sodium and potassium.

When you don't keep the levels so that the ratio stays within the range, you are going to break down and get worse. I recommend treatment of an elevated blood pressure with colonic irrigations — two a week for four weeks, one a week the next four weeks, one a month thereafter. We have not had any problem bringing down blood pressure so far. The ideal is approximately 120/60.

Breast Feeding

When you have a child, the most important thing, even before you cut the cord, is to have the child suckling the mother's breast. If not, it does not get the enzymes, and the Lactobacillus acidophilus bacteria that makes the baby's digestive system work the rest of his life. This is the most important fluid that you will ever put in your mouth. Breast feeding should be continued as long as the mother can tolerate the teeth. Two years is the end of it. That is when the digestive enzyme rennet leaves the stomach, and the child then has no business touching any milk product, including mother's milk after this age.

Some bottle-fed babies have been found to have no production of hydrochloric acid between the ages of 2 and 5 years, but it occurs commonly during the early teens to early 20s. **Why can't some women breast feed? Imbalance, not only from a hormonal standpoint but also from mineral and vitamin. We've had very little trouble if we have seen these women early.** Those ladies with small breasts can be helped; we use the mammary protomorphogens along with a regular program that we've developed (**Editor:** The program is not defined herein.). There is another product called Fortil, made by Standard Process that may be able to enlarge the breasts. One of the things in it is made from the leaves of Spanish moss, or Tillandsia (from Florida); this is the highest source of vitamin E we know of.

Breast Tumors

Women with breast tumors should get out of synthetics and nylons, because many of these tumors are nothing but congested milk ducts, and the surgeons want to do a radical mastectomy. Bruises will produce congested milk ducts. If they are only congested milk ducts, you can use castor oil packs, and there is evidence that supplemental iodine is helpful in treating breast lumps. The best iodine to use is Formula 636, or Atomidine, sold in health food stores in a dropper bottle.

Doctor to Patient

Cancer

I am an advisor to more than 300 doctors, and I guess I'm supervising about 200 cancer patients. In this cancer work, the first thing we do is blood, hair, and urine analysis to find out where we're going. We do an anthrone test, which is also known as the Navarre test, or Beard test; it checks for human chorionic gonadotropin (HCG).

I don't know of a single method that will cure all types of cancer. On most of these patients, we use about three different things and, as long as we use them together, we get somewhere. B17 (Amygdalin, Laetrile) should be legalized, if for no other reason than it is the best pain reliever in cancer patients that I know of. It's better than demerol, Darvon, or morphine. I think Dr. Philip Benzan of Washington Courthouse in Ohio has the highest cure rating with B17 by itself, and that's about 18%. Studies on germanium therapy for cancer were done by Dr. Asai in northern Japan. Dr. Asai showed us case histories and slides from 30 patients, each having been given less than two months to live, but who were all completely cancer-free after a month of treatment.

Most cure rates are down around 10-12%. Even those from Mexico are doing about the same. A lot of these organizations will say to use only B17, which we don't want. But a cancer patient also requires a very specific diet that, for the first month, allows no proteins, because we want to get away from putrefying protein. All people that I know with cancer cannot digest meat properly, so it putrefies and causes cell degeneration. They need HCl, trypsin, and chymotrypsin, in addition to a disciplined, targeted regimen. So these must be supplied, as determined by the hair, blood, and urine and so we know what and how much to use, and when.

Then we have Mitozyme, and we cannot get Dr. Lester Wesners to give us its analysis. But our analysis tells us it has a great deal of thymus in it, which of course, is one of the biggest activators of the immune response against any disease. The other thing that holds people back is that a six-week treatment is fairly expensive. But on many of these cancer patients, it does a fantastic job. However with the materials in it, you cannot use pancreatic enzymes or vitamin C, which is pretty tough on the patient. So on many of these patients, we have gone along about six to 12 weeks, either one or two rounds.

Editor: As of 2016, the product name Mitozyme is registered in India by Southern Petrochemical Industries Corporation Limited and is described as being a "Concentrate versatile enzyme preparation developed exclusively to reduce wrinkles and growth marks, imparts appreciable softness and smoothness to the leather." **It is doubtful that it is the same product mentioned in the text by Dr. Ellis.**

Then we take them off that and put them on our method with the Wobe Mugos proteolytic and pancreatic enzymes. That is the name of the German product. Here, we use Retenzyme and Intenzmye made by Biotics Research Corporation. These enzymes, by the way, if taken when an injury occurs, like a sprained ankle in sports (take five Intenzyme tablets), cut out most of the pain and swelling in about 24-48 hours. The trypsin and chymotrypsin neutralize the inflammation and swelling in the system, which has been documented with football players. We use 17 germanium tablets along with it.

I worked with the Brozny-Levinsky Clinic in Pittsburgh using Mycorrhiza. They were put out of business but came back with it as a food supplement. It does work with some people, and we have found that it works in conjunction with other things, but not too much. I worked with Dr. Bill Coate in Detroit in 1936-37 until the 1940s, when he was put on trial. We worked with glyoxalide and parabenzoquinone. Parabenzoquinone is the finest antibiotic I have used in all my years of practice and is far superior to penicillin, erythromycin, acromycin, paramycin, or any of the other mycins. One shot intramuscularly in the buttocks can usually knock out any infectious disease in the body.

Glyoxalide was synthesized by William Frederick Koch (1885-1967). It is taken intramuscularly in the buttocks. Glyoxalide increases the oxidative index of the body. It is number one on my list for treating cancers of all types. Then again, you have a specific diet that must be followed with no proteins or tomatoes. Koch taught me in his clinic, where he was treating 30-40 cancer patients of various types a day.

Glyoxalide works on a cycle of three; every three days you should have a reaction like a cold or you feel a little more tired than you were the day before, or the day after. A woman in California with cancer had to go to bed on the 21st day; she had such a reaction; on the next day, she couldn't believe how good she felt. I'd told her that anything that divides by three will give a reaction. When you multiply it in the multiples, you will get an even bigger reaction. The biggest reaction is on the 27th week. I don't know why, but this was the published routine. However if you don't get a reaction on that day then you should get another Injection of glyoxalide, to keep it in the same routine. Combined with the diet, you can get better results than anything else that I know of.

Editor: See *Virginia Livingston, M.D.: Cancer Quack or Medical Genius?* by Alan Cantwell, M.D., reprinted by permission of the author in Additional Reading on page 195.

As of 2016, it is possible to determine an individual's genetic propensity to develop certain types of cancers. The reader is encouraged to review the following website that discusses genetic tests for breast cancer: https://www.knowbrca.org/Learn/brca1-and-brca2-gene-mutations and the following website that discusses genetic tests for prostate cancer: http://time.com/4395658/aggressive-prostate-cancer-test/.

Castor Oil Versatility

Castor oil is used commonly as a laxative. However, the use of castor oil packs in any area of the body is helpful to relieve pain. Put castor oil on the affected area and cover it with a towel and apply a heating pad. Congested milk ducts in the breasts call for castor oil packs. A good book about using castor oil packs is *The Palma Christie* by William MacCary M.D. See also Eye Inflammation (Blepharitis) on page 174.

Cholesterol Elevation

Cholesterol is manufactured in the lining of the intestinal tract and liver mainly from starches, sugar, and dairy. Less than 15% is ingested, so beware of TV advertising. To lower cholesterol, eat eggs daily — a fine source of protein — just remember that under the shell is the enzyme avidin, which on exposure to the air, immediately destroys the biotin and pantothenic acid in the egg. So, I recommend that you eat eggs soft boiled for at least 30 seconds to destroy the avidin. You can eat six eggs per day and never worry about cholesterol. Supplementation may include niacin, vitamin C, and vanadium.

Chron's Disease

Chron's disease is an inflammatory bowel disease in the form of colitis. Again, you have to go with the digestive enzymes and use aloe vera gel to do the healing. The aloe vera taken by mouth does an excellent job. Raw cabbage juice (without the pulp) and lactobacillus tablets are of great help, as well. **Do not eat the cabbage pulp; it can kill you!** You may mix the aloe vera gel into the cabbage juice, or you can drink the aloe vera with cranberry or prune juice in the daytime.

If you do not have a juicer, take 1/4 head of cabbage and put it in a blender. Add one quart of distilled water, put the lid on the blender, and blend it on a high setting until the particles are as small as you can get them. Strain the mixture, discarding the pulp (again, do not eat the pulp), and store the juice in a glass bottle with a tight lid; it is very aromatic, to say the least! Drink eight ounces of this at bedtime, preferably on an empty stomach to protect the lactobacillus organisms from digestive juices.

You can also use highly concentrated chlorophyll; made from buckwheat, available from Standard Process, and the protomorphogens of the GI tract. Take each one 30 minutes before each meal; you can also use comfrey and pepsin or Hydrozyme from Biotics Research Corporation. The healing properties of these is great! Sulfa drugs are very harmful. They work for only four days, and then make your infection worse.

Colds and Flu

Whenever you have the first sign of a cold or flu, you're not up to par, you're sort of listless, and you're tired, we recommend a cleansing enema to flush putrefied, fermented, and rancid substances from the bowel. These devitalize a person, are easily eliminated, and prepare the bowel to absorb beneficial nutrients. You do this by getting from the drugstore Fleet's Phospho-Soda. On the label they tell you to take two teaspoons and a glass of water. I will tell you to take six teaspoons or two tablespoons in a glass of cold water due to the fact that this is a salt and it goes down a whole lot easier in cold water. After you put that one down, follow it with a glass of hot water as hot as you can drink it.

This is a flushing mechanism. This will flush your gallbladder and your liver and then the bile will activate your bowels completely from your stomach right on through, and especially as it gets into the small intestinal tract and empties your gallbladder of bile. Then the bile activates it in a normal and natural way. It will operate somewhere between 15 minutes and two hours. While you are waiting, take a lemon enema; that's the juice of a freshly squeezed and strained lemon in two quarts of warm water.

Deodorant Interference

What can you use for a deodorant? That's easy, don't have constipation. Because if you don't have constipation, you don't have a body odor. Why do you need any kind of deodorant; even talcum powder just blocks the pores, and you must keep them open to get rid of the extra poisons in your perspiration. The poisons should have come out of the bowel and the kidneys first. When it doesn't, it gives you a body or breath odor. Whatever you do, don't use antiperspirants that contain aluminum, because they block the third passage of elimination of poisons out of your body.

Depression

How does one combat depression? Well, the first thing anyone should do is learn how to live on a positive realm. Always look for the good out of everything, regardless of how bad it seems. Next, do the blood, hair, and urine analyses and find out where the discrepancies and metal poisonings are. When you get rid of these, there doesn't seem to be any more problems with these kinds of people. One of the things you want to realize with this type of disorder was shown in the work of Dr. Alexander Schauss, who worked in the prison systems. He found that murderers and rapists are hypoglycemic. Hypoglycemia, low blood sugar, is probably one of the most common diseases that exist today. We teach doctors that can't make a diagnosis to write down hypoglycemia, and they will be right 90% of the time. It is the greatest masquerader of all diseases that we know of.

Editor: Dr. Alexander Schauss wrote a book titled *Low Blood Sugar and Antisocial Behavior*. He explains how sugar can cause a whole range of behavioral symptoms, "from depression and hyperactivity to acting out behaviors that may be extremely asocial." Dr. Schauss uses case histories, graphs and illustrations to show the connection between food additives, food allergies, alcoholism, junk food, and environmental pollutants and how all of these contribute to the development of crime.

Diabetes

Anybody with a high blood sugar level should always check zinc, chromium, potassium, and protein to give the body the opportunity to let the glands do their job. With respect to thyroid, if you don't check the amount of inorganic iodine and the amount of protein, which are the two things blended together by the cells of the thyroid to produce thyroxine; you will never learn anything about thyroid function. The ideal ratio is 3:1. Anything over 4:1 gives hyperactivity of the thyroid gland and highly nervous, irritable factors. The same can occur even though you could have an absolutely perfect T3, T4, T8, T9, or Protein Bound Iodine (PBI).

Supplement to the deficiencies of minerals and ensure optimum protein assimilation.

Disc Degeneration

You may have disc lesions that you will never know, because they never hit a nerve root. If the rupture is through the anterior side, you never know it because there's no nerve there. We can detect it by sclerotherapy, using a 6" needle going in from the side, and directly through the disc area, using dyes and X-ray. We inject a sclerosing material and heal that ruptured disc on the inside. Then we pull it out on the outside capsular ligaments.

Once, I had a patient with a torn back, taking sclerosing treatment. I was using magnesium, but low back pain kept recurring. We started him on manganese, and this time, when he came back from his treatment, he had no more problems. Manganese is the catalyst that makes calcium, magnesium, and phosphorus do their job on the muscle and ligamentous integrity of the body. All you need is one tablet of manganese at lunch time. If you supplement yourself in calcium and magnesium, you should take calcium at or before breakfast and magnesium at dinner time.

Exercise Precautions

If you go jogging, you must make sure that you keep your body perfectly straight. If you bend forward as you jog your heart keeps hitting against your chest wall and be damaged. The men who are now jogging, standing in upright positions, instead of bending over like so many of them do, are getting better results and have more vitality than they did previously. **Some authors like Dr. George Goodheart tell you that you shouldn't jog at all; walking exercise is all you need.** In a good exercise, your heart should beat from 100-120 beats per minute over a long period of time. So, we used to tell that walking fast, swimming two miles a day, or riding a bicycle 10 miles a day will do the same thing from the standpoint of body functioning.

One thing that jogging does is destroy the protein metabolism in your muscles, and walking does not. That's why most of the long distance runners are on the thin side; they are utilizing and burning that protein out of their system, and it isn't replaced as much as it should be. Olympic team members were not allowed to touch a milk product for 48 hours before competitions, because they found out that it slowed them down too much. Actually they should never touch it an any time. To help with oxygenation of tissues and endurance, we recommend adding octacosanol to the diet, which is contained in high concentration in Viobin Wheat Germ Oil and in Biotics Research Corporation's Bioctasol Forte.

Common Health Issues

Editor: See the following link to Dr. Thomas K. Cureton's work about the use of wheat germ oil in physical training: https:// catalog.hathitrust.org/Record/ 001556016?type%5B%5D=author&lookfor%5B%5D=%22Cureton%2C%20Tho mas%20Kirk%2C%201901-%22&ft=

Eye Inflammation (Blepharitis)

For blepharitis, put one drop of raw castor oil in the eyes, four times a day. These drops burn but should be continued, because as the treatment progresses, the pain gets less and less. This could be a form of allergy, so the treatment should be continued as needed; otherwise, it can be discontinued until the next time it is necessary. We have also used the castor oil to dissolve cataracts inside the eye, using one drop four times a day.

If you wear contact lenses, get some pure castor oil and place one drop in your eyes each night before you go to bed. Close it and don't rub it. This is probably the finest healer for the conjunctiva of your eye and removes all of the irritating factors that you might get from your contact lens. Automobile mechanics or anybody working where dirt can fall into the eyes should always keep a dropper bottle of castor oil around. It is thick and stops the itching; everything rolls over to the inner corner of your eye, and it is very simple to take it out with a handkerchief.

Fasting and Congestive Heart Failure

I do not believe in fasting because unloading so much poison out into the system can create a "charley horse" in the heart muscle. One of my closest friends was George Tong. He invented the Tong Table, a really fine manipulative table. George ran the biggest health food store down in St. Louis, Missouri.) We were at an osteopathic convention when he said, "I'm going home to go on a 12-day fast." I said, "After you get through with this convention and the food that you've been eating, you'd better not do It. You will get congestive heart failure and die." That's exactly what he did. He went home, fasted, and died on the twelfth day.

I have seen this happen too many times, and that's the reason why I still say that I would rather use our other methods of detoxification, like the A and E emulsions, along with aloe vera gel. I'd rather use this slow method than a fast method. To detoxify quickly, do what I said is the equal of a 12-day fast by using sixteen grapefruit and hydrochloric acid tablets. See Fasting Alternative (Quick Grapefruit Fast) on page 108.

Fluorescent Lighting Precautions

Overhead fluorescent lights cause your brain to deteriorate. It also lowers the resistance mechanisms of your body, so don't stay under florescent lighting. I attribute the harmful effects of fluorescent lights to radiation or to the spectral balance. If you must work under these lights, wear a visor and consume foods and supplements rich in antioxidants.

Fluoride Toxicity

The federal courts in Pennsylvania and Illinois have already decided that fluorides cause cancer. I received word on toothpastes containing fluoride. They also cause cancer in your cheeks and gums. I just hope that all of these companies, the dental health associations, and the Public Health Service wake up to how dangerous fluoride is. Fluorides displace iodine in the tissues and destroy the production of hydrochloric acid in your stomach. Drink distilled water and supplement to your mineral deficiencies. Long-term consumers of fluoridated water should check the inorganic iodine and total protein levels and supplement accordingly.

Food Allergies

The top five allergenic foods are milk products, chocolate, wheat, corn, and beef, in that order. **Peanut allergy is the leading cause of anaphylaxis and death due to food allergy.** We can add to that the coal tar products — synthetic vitamins, and we can even get into it as far as metal poisonings creating an allergic reaction. The allergen swells the mucous membranes, and creates an irritation in the nose and throat area. That makes the area wide open for pollen or dust to have easy access for more irritation, because these areas are already swollen and irritated.

There are several things that help get rid of allergies. First, eliminate from your diet the things that produce allergies. Use bee pollen to stop allergies. It contains 20 of the amino acids (including all eight essentials), vitamins, and minerals. A natural antihistamine with beef liver extract is often helpful. Standard Process has a product called Antronex, containing the Japanese yakatron beef liver extract. Take one of these pills three times a day, and you will see improvements; discontinue treatment when no longer necessary.

Food Poisoning

For suspected food poisoning, hydrochloric acid is the antiseptic in the stomach. The best treatment is large doses of betaine HCl or apple cider vinegar. It either lets food progress along the tract or causes vomiting. If antibiotics are used, always follow up with Lactobacillus acidophilus and bifidus to reestablish the desired bowel flora. These bacteria help digest the fiber and avoid constipation. The emulsified vitamins A and E are helpful. Because hydrochloric acid and pepsin can destroy many protomorphogens that we ingest, select those that are prepared to withstand the acid medium until they pass into the small intestine.

Foot Strains and Sprains

There are three bones in the ankle that are always rotated and stuck; the most important one is the cuboid. The second most important is the middle cuneiform, and the third is the tibia; it always rotates posterior on the talus. **All three must be manipulated. These must be treated as soon as they occur and strapped with no inversion or eversion of the foot.** Then, one can be put back on his or her feet with no problems. Balance Is important, and if this injury is not treated, there will be a chronic ankle problem for life. Also use pancreatic enzymes to take out the inflammation and swelling.

Gout

Uric acid causes gout. People with gout are usually very low in potassium, the neutralizer for uric acid in the body. They are also very low in hydrochloric acid, and pepsin. Pork products are loaded with uric acid; they also have nitrites, nitrates, and nitrosamines, which are cancer agents. Also, don't eat sardines, because the DNA mixes with uric acid and makes the hands and feet swell. In addition to the hydrochloric acid and pepsin, use one teaspoon daily of Carbamide by Standard Process.

Hands (Cold Hands)

The hands falling asleep is an indication of a potential heart attack. The other indication is a low thyroid functioning. Cold hands and feet need ribonucleic acid, called RNA potassium, and betaine hydrochloride. These are the factors that you must put together, and you can get rid of your cold hands and feet. The only counterindication to the use of RNA is a possible rise in uric acid.

Healing of Tissues

If you are having a hard time healing, or if you are going in for surgery, take vitamin T (sesame seed factor) because it will aid in the healing process by encouraging platelet formation. Vitamin E will help to keep platelets from sticking together and aggregating. The night before surgery, have them give you a bottle of amino acids with 3,000 mg of vitamin C. We have had hundreds of patients doing this. We have no shock, no pneumonia, and they are up on the same day of surgery. Their stitches are out on the fourth day, and they go home on the fifth day.

The following lists conditions and supplementation that may restore normality to the indicated tissues. However, it is always better to determine the need for minerals based on comprehensive testing, rather than being overloaded with minerals that you may not need.

Skin conditions, including fungus (such as athletes foot), warts, etc.: Supplement with zinc, copper, and cobalt.

Nasal congestion, sore throat and mouth (including cold sores): Supplement with cobalt, manganese, magnesium, iodine, vitamins B1 and B6, emulsified vitamins A and E, and tryptophan.

Fractures: We use 20 cc of 2% magnesium chloride solution IV once weekly, with vitamin and mineral supplementation that includes copper and cobalt.

Immune system support: We use calcium lactate, vitamin F, thymus, vitamin C, and proteins.

Cardiovascular integrity: Supplement with sodium, potassium, calcium, magnesium, zinc copper, molybdenum, chromium, vanadium, manganese, iodine, and cobalt

Heart "Attack"

A true heart attack involves a problem within the heart itself. However, many deaths attributed to heart attacks may not be true heart attacks at all. Let me ask you an important question, What room in the house has the highest frequency of deaths due to heart attacks? It is the bathroom! Are you surprised? Because most people have their heart attacks within two hours after a meal; what happens is that they are not digesting their food so they get a gas pocket, either in the stomach or the transverse colon. Persons suffering from pain go to the bathroom to get an alkalizer. What happens then? After taking the alkalizer, gas in the stomach increases, causing an increase in upward pressure, stopping the diaphragm from working properly, creating severe pressure on the heart, and producing a cardiac spasm. This spasm can be so great that it can kill before relief of pressure can be obtained. When the person dies, the heart comes back to normal; they do an autopsy and can't find anything wrong with the heart.

If you ever get a chest pain up on that side, head for the kitchen and take some apple cider vinegar — one or two tablespoons in a small amount of water. Always use apple cider vinegar and drink it. If the pain is due to the gas pocket bottling up and producing a charlie horse, that acetic acid will break that bond, and you won't have a charlie horse any more, the vinegar relaxes it. It is one of the easiest tests you can give on a heart attack. **But, if that pain persists beyond five minutes you had better get somebody to get you to a hospital because you are having a heart attack.**

Heartburn

See Ulcers on page 189.

Hemorrhoids

A hemorrhoid or pile is nothing more than a varicose vein in the rectum. To relieve hemorrhoids, use aloe vera gel. Take a baby syringe containing two ounces of aloe vera gel. People that have hemorrhoids or piles should inject that solution into their rectums before they go to bed at night and let it stay there, soothing and shrinking the tissue.

Iodine Deficiency

The thyroid is not the only tissue that needs iodine; it is needed by breast, salivary, pancreas, brain, spinal fluid, skin, stomach, and thymus tissue, as well. There are two popular sources of iodine: kelp capsules and iodine solutions. There is only one kelp that anyone should use today and that comes out of Norway and it is pretty hard to get. There's plenty of American kelp, but it is pretty bad. You're also unable to ascertain with kelp the amount of iodine that your thyroid needs. Kelp, when you analyze it, varies so tremendously. I've found problems from the use of kelp. So we just tell people not to use It.

We would rather they use the Formula 636 (Atomidine). That way we know exactly what we're dealing with. You might use from one drop per week to one drop or even more per day. If a sore throat results, discontinue until the condition goes away, then resume at a lower dosage. There is evidence that supplemental iodine is helpful in treating the enlarged prostate and breast lumps. Atomidine is sold in health food stores in a dropper bottle.

Kidney Stones

A kidney problem signals a bowel problem, because most of the body's poisons are supposed to be going into the bowel. When the bowel can't handle these poisons, they go to the kidneys. This insult is in addition to what the kidney itself has to do. Most of these are caused by the urine being too alkaline, again a lack of hydrochloric acid and pepsin. The sodium and potassium must be in balance to make the kidneys work properly. The pH is very important because most kidney infections or diseases occur in an alkaline urine.

Any pains in the kidneys, ureters, bladder, and urethra are more severe when the urine is alkaline. Many times, you can relieve such pain with just a couple of teaspoons of vinegar. You might need to form antibodies to fight the infections, and then acidify them. You can clear up most of them in this manner.

For calcium stones, we use phosphorus and magnesium, dissolving the calcium stones and enabling them to be passed. We then use a big dose of olive oil or castor oil. The hardest ones to clear up are uric acid stones, which can form in the kidneys or gallbladder. They can be removed surgically without having to take the kidney or gallbladder out.

To lessen the chance of developing stones, the vegetables In salads, such as cabbage, cauliflower, spinach, and tomatoes, should always be eaten raw; never cooked. They are all high in oxalic acid, which interferes with calcium metabolism. The only fruit that leave an acid residue are prunes, plums, cranberries, and rhubarb. Rhubarb should be eaten raw because of its oxalic acid content. All other fruits leave an alkaline residue (make the urine alkaline). When you eat alkaline fruit, it is much better to eat them as a snack individually between meals, at least three hours after protein.

Knee Joint Deterioration

What can be done for the deterioration of the knee that is causing pain and fluid buildup? The first thing would be to examine it for a rotation of the tibia on the femur. I did this for one of the football players for the Buffalo Bills. They asked me to take a look at it. This player had been in constant pain for two years and yet was playing football. He came over to my hotel room. When I travel, I always carry my portable table with me. I set it up, put him on the table, and there was this rotation. So, instead of coming through even when he turned, it would hit and irritate. He started getting an inflammation in the knee.

I pump handled it a little while and stretched the cartilages that had not been operated on, because he had had two operations on one knee, and one on the other. It took me about 10 minutes of doing this on the two knees on each side. I got him up, and we walked up and down the room. He said, "I can't believe it, I am walking for the first time in two years with absolutely no pain." We recommend using emulsified cod liver oil on a long-term basis. See Arthritis on page 164.

Liver Toxicity

Let's go over how to detoxify the liver. Number one, take vitamin A, vitamin F, and beet juice extract from Standard Process 30 minutes before a meal. This will thin the bile and let it flow. That's the easiest and fastest way to get it out. The use of aloe vera gel by taking two to four ounces every day gives you the opportunity of healing the gastrointestinal tract, and making it flow better. Coffee enemas do the same thing. But probably the great thing you need the most is hydrochloric acid, and pepsin within the stomach. Because if you don't have sufficient amounts of hydrochloric acid, the liver does not do its job. Neither does the bile come out of the gallbladder as it should.

Chew your food thoroughly to take the strain off your liver and intestinal tract, because if you don't have enough enzymes, you're going to putrefy the protein and ferment the starches and sugars. The end products have to be filtered through the liver, and if you don't have sufficient digestion, you are going to clog the liver. Let's predict, prevent, and keep out of trouble from the start. If a cleansing is necessary, follow the appropriate procedures given in Detoxification on page 97.

Lupus and Other Autoimmune Conditions

We have had some success with lupus, but not total success. We use the same type of treatment as for malignant conditions. See Cancer on page 168.

Menstrual Problems

Many women with menstrual problems have a cholesterol level that is too low. They are treated by having them eat more fats; their ovaries produce more hormones and get rid of dysmenorrhea or menopausal hot flashes. In our diet, we require both saturated and unsaturated fats. Foods to eat are fish (as recommended previously); olive, safflower, and sunflower oils; nuts; and seeds. Cook meat at 138° F and the saturated fats will be fine.

Ladies wearing three-, four-, and five-inch heels will wind up with menstrual problems, most likely ending with a hysterectomy. The treatment for the resulting dysmenorrhea is to decrease the heel height and use what we call a knee to chest breathing exercise, which lets the uterus go forward again. Another way to get the uterus to go forward is to get pregnant and, immediately after delivery, have the mother sleep face down.

Supplementation

I use Vitaminerals formulas 2BG and Number 16. Vitaminerals 2BG has double the amounts of D complex with its mineral synergists and also contains vitamins A, B, C, and F with their mineral synergists. Number 16, a polymineral, has 34 minerals in it, and two tablets are suggested per meal.

Editor: The Vitamineral (VMMedical) Company website is currently http://www.vmmedical.com/.

Knee to Chest Breathing Exercise for Dysmenorrhea

Women have a constant small opening that runs through the vagina and cervix into the uterus, then through the fallopian tubes and up into the abdominal cavity. The objective of this exercise is to get air to suck in and out of this opening, allowing the fallopian tubes to open up. The action causes the uterus to tip over to a forward position.

Directions:

1. Start out with the woman on her back with her knees bent and feet flat on the floor.

2. Bring one knee to the chest and hold the position for 15-30 seconds. Breathe deeply, allowing the abdomen to move freely.

3. Return to the starting position.

4. Repeat the movement with the other leg.

5. Perform this exercise 2-4 times with each leg.

Metal Jewelry Irritation

Wearing metal jewelry next to your skin is harmful, and the most harmful place to wear metal is the midline of the body; this is especially true for glasses. The presence of metal upsets the electrical field of the body. One half of your brain has a positive magnetic charge, the other half a negative magnetic charge. If you have metal in the middle line you neutralize brain function. If you have a big belt buckle in the midline, being the location of your solar plexus, it destroys the function of the nerves of the solar plexus. So never wear metal on the midline, put it on one side or the other.

Now one thing we know, if you put on certain things like copper bracelets or anklets it can be good for you, or it can be harmful to you. **One should do a hair analysis to find out what minerals are imbalanced in the tissues before attempting to wear a copper bracelet.** If you have too much copper in your system and put a copper bracelet on, it will break down your brain, your nerves, and your blood vessels. It is important that you neutralize, normalize, and make everything in balance; then you will not have any problems.

Multiple Sclerosis

One of the things we have found in most multiple sclerosis cases is metal poisoning, with aluminum being number one on the list. We try to neutralize these metals, using octacosanol, superoxide dismutase (SOD), and catalase. These have been used very successfully.

There was an experienced physician in a veterans hospital who took six of the M. S. cases and used octacosanol, superoxide dismutase, and catalase; he was getting very good results. What do you think happened? They transferred him out of the division so he couldn't touch the cases any more. That's what you run into with the kind of medicine we see from the American Medical Association. If you take SOD straight it does form peroxides. But if you use catalase to neutralize the peroxides, it's a very excellent product. We use it to normalize cell development and cell function. Catalase is found in all normal cells, but most people don't have enough, so we give it to them to rebuild the cell structures.

Muscle Pulls (Charlie Horses)

You can put double-wide pieces of non-waterproof tape above and below a pulled muscle to keep the pull from spreading. During walking or running, the tape becomes a massaging agent. You may expect the pull to become smaller at the end of the activity.

Always remove the tape in the evening; this is especially important in persons with fair skin. Do not have any tape on for more than 48 hours. Check the blood calcium level, the calcium/phosphorus ratio and the level of manganese in the system, if possible.

Osteoporosis

Someone asked me, "What would you advise the older ladies with osteoporosis to do?" We suggest doing 44 blood tests, 19 metals in the hair, a standard urinalysis, and the patient's seven-day diet. Then we analyze and correlate the results to find out what may be causing the osteoporosis, among many other possibilities. Osteoporosis comes from a lack of the balance of the minerals, mainly calcium, magnesium, manganese, and phosphorous. It also is a hormonal insufficiency; thus you see this in the older people. If you don't have sufficient hormones, it is one of your biggest problems in rheumatoid arthritis, along with imbalances of those four minerals. It is the variance of the ratios among each of these that helps to produce this type of disease.

Editor: John D. Carter, MD is the Director of Clinical Research for the Division of Rheumatology at the University of South Florida. His primary research focuses on Chlamydia-induced Reactive Arthritis. **Chlamydia trachomatis is the leading sexually-transmitted bacterial infection in the United States and can cause a serious form of arthritis (reactive arthritis, or ReA) in some individuals.** Chlamydial infections can also exist in a persistent state that has been linked to not only ReA, but also other potential diseases. It is believed to play a role in some of the adverse effects that occur with certain treatments for other types of arthritis. Practitioners treating arthritis, osteoporosis, and spondylitis should review the following of Dr. Carter's publications.

Carter JD, Valeriano J, Vasey FB. *A Prospective, Randomized 9-Month Comparison of Doxycycline vs. Doxycycline and Rifampin in Undifferentiated Spondyloarthropathy - with Special Reference to Chlamydia-Induced Arthritis. Journal of Rheumatology.* 31(10):1973-80, 2004.

Carter JD, Valeriano J, Vasey FB. *Antimicrobials for the Treatment of Chlamydia-Induced Reactive Arthritis. Annals of the Rheumatic Diseases.* 64(3):512-3, 2005.

Carter, JD, Espinoza LR. *The Interplay of Environment and Host Response in Reactive Arthritis: Can We Intervene? Future Rheumatology.* 1(6):717-27, 2006.

Parasites

Ninty percent of people have parasites. The feeling is almost like the flu. Again we go to blood work to determine whether parasites are present in the system. The following story will illustrate what I am trying to tell you.

I had a radiologist call me from Atlanta, Georgia. He said, "Doctor for two years I have been trying to find out what is wrong with me. I weighed 190 pounds, and now I weigh 100. I have been to the best doctors in this entire area trying to find out what is wrong with me. Nobody knows what it is. I was just talking to a friend of yours, and he says you are the best diagnostician in the country and that I'd better call you on the phone." I said, "Well doctor, I imagine your being a doctor yourself that you have done some blood chemistry work; let's start with your CBC, the complete blood count."

White blood count: normal is 5-10,000, ideal 7,500; his was 3,200. His red cell count was down to 3,200, this means that he was anemic. Hemoglobin for men should be between 15 and 16; his was 13.2. The hematocrit, which indicates the volume of a red blood cell, was also pathologic; the cells were too small. The normal count for eosinophils is 1-3, he had 70. Then we looked at the count, and I asked what was it four or five? He said, "Five."

I said," I know what's wrong with you. You have got parasites, microorganisms, or worms." He said, "But doctor, I had a stool culture, and they didn't find anything." I said, "Doctor, do you think that worms can be only in the intestinal tract?" He said, "Yes." I said, "Man, you have got a lot of studying to do." We find these in the brain, in the muscles, heart, tissues; you name it, and we have found them. You are loaded with them."

Chickens and turkeys that are raised on wire are loaded with a microorganism called Progenitor cryptocides (see Additional Reading on page 195). These are part of the microorganisms we are talking about. So, always check whether the chicken or the turkey that you are about to buy were raised on the ground. If not, don't buy them.

We can get rid of these microorganisms in several ways. The fast way, which can also cause reactions, is to take a half a teaspoon of confectionary sugar. On this, put six drops of turpentine and swallow it. Man, does it react. Do this at night, then the next morning either take a dose of Fleets Phospho-Soda or a couple teaspoons of castor oil, and some prune juice; then you don't taste it at all. That will really take them out of your system in a hurry.

There is a milder way of doing this. Standard Process has two things one can use. The first is called Zymex II, and the second is called Multizyme. We use Zymex II more than we use anything. Take three of them four times a day for three weeks, and then you cut them to one three times a day for another month. We usually get rid of the parasites in that period of time.

Prostate Problems

Supplemental iodine is helpful in treating the enlarged prostate, as well as other prostate conditions. The best iodine to use is Formula 636 (Atomadine), sold in health food stores in a dropper bottle. You might use from one drop per week to one drop or even more per day. If a sore throat results, discontinue until the condition goes away, then resume at a lower dosage.

Psoriasis

Psoriasis is cholesterol coming out of the pores of your skin. Lower your cholesterol and you'll find it's what we are doing today with emulsions of RNA-DNA, hydrochloric acid, and the pancreatic enzymes, we are clearing up probably most of these in 6 to 8 weeks. Apply Borage oil topically.

Sciatica

See Back Pain (Lower Back/Anatomical Short Leg) on page 164.

Shoulder Pain

When I went over to see the Buffalo Bills football team, I treated six of them, including one of their officers, who said, "What do you do for shoulders, I can't get my arms up any higher than this." I said, "Jump up here on this table." This guy had an anterior third rib out in the front. The one on the left side controls 16 organs, and 22 muscles. The one on the right side, 8 organs, and 22 muscles. I fixed this rib first. Then, I did the pump handle on his elbows and then his shoulders. I corrected the acromio-clavicular lesion, that's where the collar bone is in the shoulder joint. Where we see rib and disc lesions all of the time is with an anatomical short leg. It causes a twist in the knee, the back, or the shoulders as well as up into the head. It also can give you headaches. Take trypsin and chymotrypsin supplements to reduce inflammation.

Skin Conditions

To keep the skin nice and flexible; take vitamin A and E emulsions each day. Routinely do blood analysis and hair mineral analysis every year and supplement for deficiencies. The emulsions, along with Lactobacillus acidophilus and bifidus, draining the liver and gallbladder, and stimulating the adrenals, produce anti-inflammatory agents. With proper diet, the skin condition should clear up in six weeks. Add the thyroid protomorphogen (Standard Process Thyrotropin) to clear up psoriasis; remember that thyroid function and cholesterol levels are inversely related. People with skin diseases must be detoxified, according to the protocols listed in Detoxification on page 97. The key is to keep your body balanced. Postural balance is of key importance too. Add omega 3 oils to your diet.

Stroke

The main cause of strokes is arterio- or atherosclerosis. One of the important factors are the triglycerides — today considered more important than cholesterol. Oranges will raise triglycerides faster than anything else I know of. Other foods that cause a rise in blood triglycerides are processed starches, sugars, and milk products. These must be avoided. Treatment and physical therapy will be tailored to the patient, based on the severity of clinical symptoms. Adjuncts to treatment may involve lowering triglycerides with vitamin C, thinning the blood with HCl in the diet, dilating the blood vessels with vitamin B3, and strengthening the vessel walls with vitamin E, but care must be taken not to interfere with prescribed medications.

Sunburn (Tendency to Sunburn)

I believe that the tendency to sunburn is influenced by the level of calcium in the body. Brunettes are low in calcium, and blonds and redheaded persons are especially low. Supplement calcium if you have a tendency to burn and not tan well. Use all sensible precautions to avoid too much exposure to the sun, and keep in mind that you can burn just as severely on an overcast day.

Teeth Fragility and Pain

To have good teeth, start early in life, stay away from all starches, sugars, and milk products. One of the worst cavity producers is cheese. One of the most severe causes of migraine headaches that we know of is the phenylethylamine in cheese. Taken together, all milk products are the single greatest cause of disease in the human body that I know of.

Painful teeth need magnesium, zinc, iodine, and methionine. Along with these trace elements, methionine can cause the gums to grow back along the tooth and maintain a very tight attachment at the gingival margin. It was shown by Dr. Ralph Steinman many years ago how completely permeable the teeth are to iodine.

Dental Caries (Cavities)

In 1919, Melvin E. Page, D.D.S. began practicing dentistry in Muskegon, Michigan and soon became known as a top prosthodontist. He noticed that it was necessary to remake the classic dentures for many of his patients within two and a half years. Their jaw bones would resorb under the dentures and bridges. To learn why his patients' mouths deteriorated, Dr. Page ran more than 2,000 blood chemistries. **He found that no absorption of bone and no cavities occurred when the blood calcium to phosphorus ratio (Ca/P) was in a proportion of 10 to 4, or 2.5:1. Dr. Page also found that the blood sugar level should be at 85, plus or minus 5 (Sclavo test) and that resorption of bone would stop when the Ca/P ratio was restored to 2.5.** He also cautioned against eating white sugar and refined carbohydrates and drinking milk. He advocated the use of vitamin and mineral supplements and the avoidance of chemical additives and preservatives in foods.]

Editor: Thanks to the International Foundation for Nutrition and Health for the information about Dr. Page. For further information about the IFNH, see http://ifnh.org/product-category/educational-materials/pioneers-of-nutrition/dr-melvin-e-page.

Environment of the Mouth

The mouth should be isoelectric, meaning there should be no electrical current activity occurring within. The presence of mercury amalgam fillings allows such activity to occur. Major acupuncture circuits go through the teeth as follows:

- The upper and lower central lateral incisors relate to the kidney and urinary bladder.
- The cuspids relate to the liver and gallbladder.
- The lower molars and upper premolars relate the the large intestine and lung.
- The lower bicuspids and upper molars relate to the spleen, pancreas, and stomach.
- The third molars relate to the heart and small intestines.
- Each tooth is also related to the function of nine muscles.

When electrical conductivity occurs across the teeth, all of the endocrine glands are affected adversely. Also, it has been shown that mercury leeches from amalgam fillings over time, subjecting the individual to varying degrees of mercury toxicity. Symptoms of mercury escaping from tooth fillings may include the following.

- Sensitivity or allergy to any metal, food, detergent, pollen, etc.
- Metallic taste in the mouth
- Burning sensation in the mouth
- Increased flow of saliva
- Gum disorder or disease
- Frequent unexplained fatigue
- Headaches
- Ringing or noise in the ears
- Cold hands or feet
- Skin rash or dermatitis
- Any change in health after dental work
- Nervous disorders in any part of the body, such as numbness, tingling, shaking, or trembling

Thyroid Deficiency

You can be harmed by taking synthroid; it is a synthetic thyroid, as is proroid, neither of which we recommend. If you are going to use thyroid itself, I would use only as a last resort. We would prefer to let the gland do its own job. We would rather use the protomorphogens of Standard Process or the neonatals of Biotics Research Corporation. The regrowth factors are made from thyroid; you use it with iodine and protein because these are the two ingredients that make thyroxine. In doing this, we are able to build the patient's thyroxine to where it belongs, and in doing so, promote normal thyroid functioning. See Iodine Deficiency on page 178.

TMJ (Temporomandibular Joint, Jaw) Pain

The temporomandibular joints are directly in front of the ears. 43% of the nervous system is connected to the TMJ. Likewise, the teeth and entirety of the mouth receive an abundant nerve supply out of proportion to the rest of the body. The teeth are related through meridians and nerves to the 12 cranial nerves, and each tooth is directly or indirectly related to a specific organ of the body. So, it is not surprising that fillings can cause neurologic allergies or irritations to all 12 of the cranial nerves.

Symptoms of irritation of the TMJ may include the following.
- Pain in the ears, including the middle and inner ear, earache, and tinnitis
- Backaches, scoliosis, neck problems, headaches, sinusitis
- Weak muscles and disequilibrium
- Pain in the shoulders
- Leg length abnormalities
- Stomach, small intestine, and endocrine abnormalities

Tranquilizer Precautions

If you want to use wonderful tranquilizers, take magnesium and vitamin B6. They are the finest tranquilizers we have ever used. They are so superior to librium or valium. Last year there were 22 million prescriptions written for valium and librium in the United States. Number one and number two on the list of all prescribed items, and all they do is destroy your liver and your kidneys.

Ulcers

Your stomach, lined with a mucous membrane, is made to hold an acid. No one has an overabundance of stomach acid; it is likely that no one has enough. See *Acid Indigestion: Myth and Mysteries, Time Magazine*, Friday, Aug. 28, 1964. **This article documents that there is no such thing as an overacid stomach.** When you age, you start losing hydrochloric acid, nature has its own way of compensating for it by regurgitating the concentrated, highly alkaline bile back into the stomach.

How They Develop

Bile burns mucous membranes and produces a gastric ulcer. If you lack hydrochloric acid in the stomach, bile will be regurgitated into the stomach. The average stomach withstands a pH of 2. The mucous membranes are made to withstand acids. Bile is highly alkaline and burns worse than acid. The constant reflux of bile causes gastritis and finally an ulcer. When we stop the bile reflux by taking hydrochloric acid, the ulcer has an opportunity to heal. Alternately, the constant irritation can lead to oversecretion of hydrochloric acid. After the food leaves the stomach, extra acid continues to be produced. The mucous membranes of the duodenum normally withstand alkalis, not acids. This hypersecretion of hydrochloric acid produces a duodenal ulcer.

A person who has had a gallbladder removed has a constant flow of bile and must be very careful about what he eats. Otherwise that bile, with no food coming through, will irritate and cause a gas problem, duodenitis, or jejunitis. Also, taking too much aspirin is one of the best ways I know to get a gastric ulcer. Being an achlorhydric, I have had to be very careful about what foods and supplements I take, so I can stay alive. If I were unable to do this, I would be in real trouble. Achlorhydrics are absolutely fit candidates for cancer. Their alpha-2-globulin and pancreatic enzyme levels are abnormal.

If a gastric ulcer is removed surgically, the problem that caused it remains. I have seen cases of gastrectomy where two-thirds of the stomach is removed from an achlorhydric. However, two months later the problems recurred. These people may not have as much acute pain, but only the symptoms have been removed. People having recurrent ulcers and on a Sippy diet (milk products) can develop new types of ulcers.

The article, *The Incidence of Coronary Heart Disease in Patients Treated with the Sippy Diet, American Journal of Clinical Nutrition*, 15:205, 1964, explains how the Sippy diet uses milk, cream, butter, eggs, and mild cheeses to treat ulcers. It is the biggest cause of strokes, and heart attacks that we know of. It never cures the ulcer, but it just creates enough mucus to cover the crater. You get rid of the symptoms, you don't feel as much pain, and you think you have done pretty good.

In one case, we had to remove the stomach of a man who had had nine ulcers. We dissected it, and right beside each area of scar tissue was a new ulcer. He had hemorrhaged so badly that we couldn't do anything else but operate. When this man healed, the first thing I had to do was teach him how to balance his lack of hydrochloric acid for the rest of his organs to work properly.

How They Can Be Healed

Ulcers are easy to clear up; I've cleared up more ulcers by giving patients hydrochloric acid and pepsin to help digest their food than any other method I've ever used. We use Standard Process comfrey and pepsin. The only thing I can tell you is that aloe vera gel is a great treatment for ulcers, and we give patients a teaspoonful at a time, every three or four hours, and we do get healing.

Pepsin is the main stimulator for the cells to make more acid. When we feel the tissue has healed sufficiently, we switch to hydrochloric acid therapy. This is how I healed my own duodenal ulcer. I have tried the same technique on others, and I have never had to resort to surgery.

Another good treatment for ulcers is to take a four- to six-ounce glass of raw cabbage juice (fresh, not canned); drink this every couple of hours all day, consuming the juice within seven minutes of extraction; the enzymes will heal the ulcer (believe me, it has a horrible aroma). Eat bland foods along with it. Do not eat the cabbage pulp itself, it could kill you!

If you do not have a juicer, take 1/4 head of cabbage and put it in a blender. Add one quart of distilled water, put the lid on the blender, and blend it on a high setting until the particles are as small as you can get them. Strain the mixture, discarding the pulp. Drink eight ounces of this at bedtime, preferably on an empty stomach.

You can also use highly concentrated chlorophyll made from buckwheat, available from Standard Process, and the protomorphogens of the GI tract. Take each 30 minutes before each meal; you can also use comfrey and pepsin or Hydrozyme from Biotics Research Corporation. Ulcers in the digestive system should heal themselves within six weeks.

Vaccination Precaution

I do not recommend vaccinations; they are not necessary, unless you want some degenerative diseases to appear in life later on. The National Health Federation has a kit that will show to you, and all authorities, that vaccinations are not necessary, and they do more harm than good. I'll tell you one thing that you learn about vaccinations like small pox. This has always been interesting to me. We haven't had it in our country for a good many years.

Weight Control Problem

With regard to the diet for obese patients, there seems to be a lot of confusion about low calories and low carbohydrates. **When you want to count calories, whatever your perfect weight is, you need 10 times the amount of calories per day.** For instance, if you weigh 150 pounds, you need 1,500 calories per day to maintain that weight.

People go to Weight Watchers and take a 500-calorie diet, thinking that they will lose weight automatically, but they will lose it at the expense of their health. **Balance your diet, staying away from the extra starches and sugars and milk products, they're the biggest ones that give you weight. If you eat raw green and yellow vegetables, rare meats, raw nuts, and seeds, this will automatically balance your diet. If you're overweight, you will lose. If you're underweight you will gain.**

Sources of proteins? Meat, fresh eggs, fish, and gelatin are your best sources of protein. The fish is the top of protein that you can buy; I recommend salt water fish. The only thing that you have to watch in salt water fish is the potential for lead and mercury poisoning that you can detect with the hair analysis.

Do not touch bottom fish; that includes lobster, shrimp, crabs, oysters, clams, etc. You can eat fish that stay near the surface, like tuna, salmon, sardines, etc. If you eat a can of sardines every day, it's one of the greatest helpful protein you can eat. But these are short sardines from Norway, which are loaded with natural DNA. Most of the sardines that you get are wider and longer, but they are actually herring. Now we get the natural DNA and RNA from herring sperm.

This is the poor man's cell therapy that rebuilds cell structures in the body. The only contraindications for the use of RNA-DNA is a high uric acid count in the blood, which may cause the hands and feet to swell up. What is involved in gout besides uric acid? Gout results from the inability to digest protein. Low potassium is another factor. it is the neutralizer of uric acid in the body. Supplementing hydrochloric acid and potassium can reestablish the balance.

Yeast Infections

One other thing, especially in women that we check, and that is for budding, yeast in the urine. We are seeing more and more yeast infections in women. And for the women: get away from the synthetics and the nylons especially with panty hose because they are one of the greatest mediums you have for growing a yeast infection within the vagina because they don't breathe.

Withdraw sugars from the yeast; this is best done with the healthy diet described elsewhere in this book. There are some effective herbal combinations that discourage the growth of yeast, and the lactobacillus is desirable to repopulate the intestine with beneficial bacteria that can out compete the yeast.

Common Health Issues

Appendix A: Additional Reading

Editor: This appendix contains articles and abstracts of articles related to points made by Dr. Ellis in previous chapters. **The opinions stated therein belong solely to the authors and may not all be congruent with the beliefs of Dr. Ellis, but they may shed light on the rationale that Dr. Ellis used in formulating some of his opinions.** Again, anyone afflicted with a serious disorder should seek a thorough evaluation by a licensed health practitioner and follow sound medical advice.

We thank Dr. Alan Cantwell for permission to print the following article in its entirety. Dr. Ellis held Dr. Livingston in high regard, and he believed that bacterial organisms in intracellular form were causative agents for many diseases and likely provided a focus for cancer in various tissues, unless treated and eradicated.

Dr. Alan Cantwell is a retired dermatologist and the author of *The Cancer Microbe* and *Four Women Against Cancer*, both available from Aries Rising Press, PO Box 29532, Los Angeles, CA 90029 (www.ariesrisingpress.com). Email: alancantwell@sbcglobal.net. Abstracts of 30 published papers can be found at the PubMed website (type in Cantwell AR). Many of his personal writings can be found on www.google.com by using key words "alan cantwell" + articles. His books are also available on www.amazon.com and through Book Clearing House @ 1-800-431-1579.

Virginia Livingston, M.D.: Cancer Quack or Medical Genius?

by Alan Cantwell, M.D., Los Angeles, California

Cancer is the most frightening human disease and its cause remains elusive. Therefore, it seems inconceivable that the discovery of a germ cause of cancer would provoke such hostility among the cancer establishment. But, in truth, the belief in a cancer germ has always been the ultimate scientific heresy.

In the long history of cancer research there was never a physician more outspoken and controversial than Virginia Wuerthele-Caspe Livingston (1906-1990). For more than 40 years, she championed the revolutionary idea that bacteria caused cancer and devised a treatment to try and combat these microbes by immunotherapy.

Sixteen years after her death she is now largely forgotten but still condemned by such powerful organizations as the American Cancer Society and blacklisted on Quackwatch, a self-proclaimed "non-profit corporation dedicated to combating health-related frauds, myths, fads, and fallacies."

Livingston's Cancer Research

Beginning in the late 1940s, Livingston was able to grow bacteria from cancer tumors; and when she and her associates injected cancer bacteria into laboratory animals, some developed cancer. Other animals developed degenerative and proliferative diseases, and some animals remained healthy. Livingston believed the "immunity" of the host was an important factor in determining whether cancer would develop.

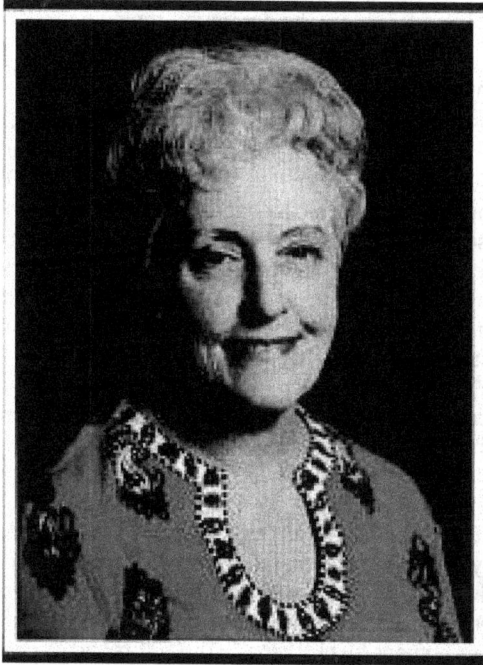

Figure 6: Virginia Livingston M.D. (1906–1990)

In 1969 at a meeting at the New York Academy of Sciences, Livingston and her colleagues proposed that cancer was caused by a highly unusual bacterium which she named Progenitor cryptocides, Greek for "ancestral hidden killer." Nevertheless, Livingston claimed elements of the microbe were present in every human cell. Due to its biochemical properties, she believed the organism was responsible for initiating life and for the healing of tissue and for killing us with cancer and other infirmities. Critics of this research continued to insist there was no such thing as a cancer germ.

In her attempt to use a variety of modalities (diet, supplements, antibiotics, as well as traditional methods) to treat cancer, she utilized an 'autogenous' vaccine derived from the patient's own cancer bacteria found in the urine and blood. Livingston explained it was not an anti-cancer vaccine, but rather a vaccine to stimulate and improve the patient's own immune system. The administration of this unapproved vaccine caused a furor in the cancer establishment and eventually legal action was undertaken against her and the Livingston-Wheeler Clinic in San Diego. In spite of all her legal troubles, she continued seeing patients until her death at 83.

In March 1990, the year of her death, a highly critical article on the Livingston-Wheeler therapy appeared in the American Cancer Society-sponsored CA: A Cancer Journal for Physicians. (No authors were listed.) The report advised patients to stay away from the San Diego clinic and claimed: "Livingston-Wheeler's cancer treatment is based on the belief that cancer is caused by a bacterium she has named Progenitor cryptocides. Careful research using modern techniques, however, has shown that there is no such organism and that Livingston-Wheeler has apparently mistaken several different types of bacteria, both rare and common, for a unique microbe. In spite of diligent research to isolate a cancer-causing microorganism, none has been found. Similarly, Livingston-Wheeler's autologous vaccine cannot be considered an effective treatment for cancer. While many oncologists have expressed the hope that someday a vaccine will be developed against cancer, the cause(s) of cancer must be determined before research can be directed toward developing a vaccine. The rationale for other facets of the Livingston-Wheeler cancer therapy is similarly faulty. No evidence supports her contention that cancer results from a defective immune system, that a whole-foods diet restores immune system deficiencies, that ascorbic acid slows tumor growth, or that cancer is transmitted to humans by chickens." (The full report is on-line at: http://caonline.amcancersoc.org/cgi/reprint/40/2/103.)

Bacteria As a Cause of Cancer

The recognition of disease-producing bacteria allowed medical science to emerge from the dark ages into the era of modern medicine. In the late nineteenth century when diseases like tuberculosis (TB), syphilis, and leprosy were proven to be caused by bacteria, some doctors also suspected human cancer might have a similar cause.

The idea that bacteria cause cancer is considered preposterous by most physicians. However, despite the antagonistic view of the American Cancer Society and medical science, there is ample evidence in the published peer-reviewed literature that strongly suggests that "cancer microbes" cause cancer.

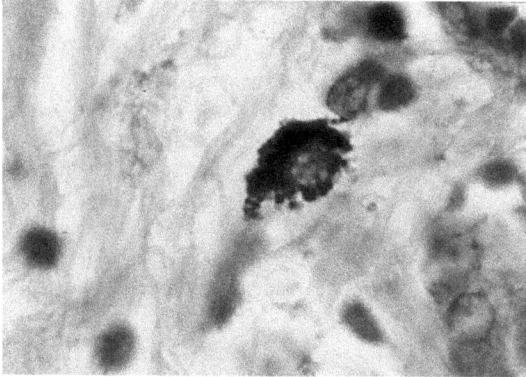

Figure 7:   Intracellular variably–sized coccoid forms in breast cancer. Acid–fast; x1,000.

According to reports by Livingston and various other researchers, cancer is caused by pleomorphic, cell wall-deficient bacteria. The various forms of the organism range in size from submicroscopic virus-like forms, up to the size of bacteria, yeasts, and fungi. In culture and in tissue the bacterial forms are variably 'acid-fast' (having a staining quality like TB bacteria). These bacteria are ubiquitous and exist in the blood and tissues of all human beings (yet another "heresy"). In the absence of a protective immune response, these cell wall-deficient bacteria may become pathogenic and foster the development of cancer, autoimmune disease, AIDS, and certain other chronic diseases of unknown etiology.

Needless to say, all of this research fell on dead ears because bacteria were totally ruled out as the cause of all cancers in the early years of the twentieth century. Thus, bacteria observed in cancer were simply dismissed as elements of cellular degeneration, or as invaders of tissue weakened by cancer, or as 'contaminants' of laboratory origin.

Livingston and Progenitor Cryptocides

Beginning in 1950, in a series of papers and books, Livingston and her co-workers claimed the cancer microbe was a great imitator whose various pleomorphic forms resembled common staphylococci, diphtheroids, fungi, viruses, and host cell inclusions. Yet if the germ were studied carefully through all its transitional stages, it could be identified as a single agent.

She was the first to suggest that the acid-fast stain was the key to the identification of the cancer microbe in tissue and in culture; and also demonstrated its appearance in the blood of cancer patients, by use of dark-field microscopy.

Anyone who takes the time to read Livingston's reports in the medical literature will quickly recognize that she was a credible research scientist, who allied herself with other experts-and was certainly not the quack doctor pictured by her detractors. Her achievements in cancer microbiology can also be found in her autobiographical books: Cancer, A New Breakthrough (1972); The Microbiology of Cancer (1977); and The Conquest of Cancer (1984). Her research has been confirmed by other scientists, such as microbiologist Eleanor Alexander-Jackson, cell cytologist Irene Diller, biochemist Florence Seibert, and dermatologist Alan Cantwell, among others.

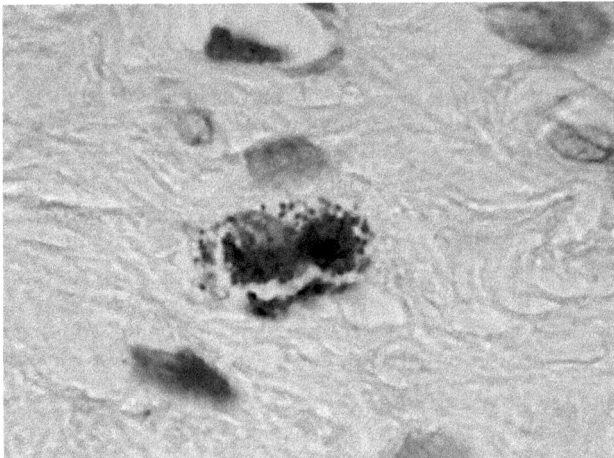

Figure 8:   Intracellular bacteria in prostate cancer.
Acid–fast; x1,000,

The Cancer Microbe and Bacterial Pleomorphism

Microbiologists have long resisted the idea of bacterial pleomorphism, and do not recognize or accept the various growth forms and the bacterial 'life cycle' proposed by various cancer microbe workers. Most bacteriologists do not accept the idea of a bacterium changing from a coccus to a rod, or to a fungus. Depending on the environment, the microbe in its cell wall-deficient phase may attain large size, even larger that a red blood cell. Other forms are submicroscopic and virus-sized. Electronic microscopic studies and photographs of filtered (bacteria-free) cultures of the cancer microbe show virus-size elements of the cancer microbe that can revert into bacterial-sized microbes.

The cancer microbe has adapted to life in man and animals by existing in a mycoplasma-like or cell wall-deficient state. In tissue sections of cancer stained for bacteria with the special acid-fast stain, the microbe can be seen as a variably acid-fast (blue, red, or purple-stained) round coccus or as barely visible granules. At magnifications of one thousand times (in oil), these forms can be observed within and also outside of the cells.

Careful study and observation of the tiny round coccoid forms in cancer tissue indicate they can enlarge progressively up to the size of so-called Russell bodies, which are well-known to pathologists. Russell bodies can attain the size of red blood cells, and even larger.

William Russell was a well-respected Scottish pathologist who in 1890 first reported the finding of 'cancer parasites' in the tissue of all of the cancers he studied. However, modern pathologists deny that Russell's bodies are microbial in origin. For more information on Russell bodies and Russell's 'cancer parasite' (and its intimate relationship to cancer microbes), Google: The forgotten clue to the bacterial cause of cancer; or go to: http:// www.joimr.org/phorum/read.php?f=2&i=50&t=50.

Overlooking Hidden Bacteria in Cancer

Once bacteria were eliminated as a cause of cancer a century ago, it became dogma and impossible to change medical opinion. In this current era of medical science, one would think it impossible for infectious disease experts and pathologists to not recognize bacteria in cancer. However, bacteria can still pop up in diseases in which they were initially overlooked.

When a new and deadly lung disease broke out among legionnaires in Philadelphia in July 1976, 222 people became ill and 34 died. The cause of the killer lung disease remained a medical mystery for over five months until Joe McDade at the Leprosy Branch of the CDC detected unusual bacteria in guinea pigs experimentally infected with lung tissue from the dead legionnaires. Further modification of bacterial culture methods finally allowed the isolation of the causative and previously overlooked bacteria, now known as Legionella pneumophila.

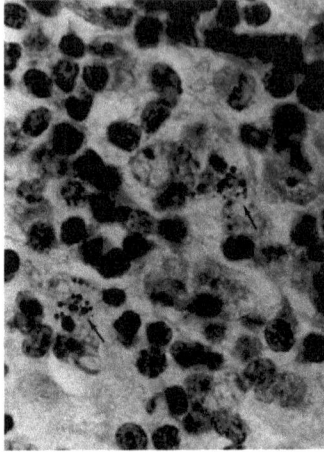

Figure 9: Lymph node showing Hodgkin's lymphoma. Gram stain; x1,000.

Arrows point to variably-sized round coccoid forms and larger Russell bodies.

Yet another example of dogma-defying research is provided by recent studies proving that bacteria (Helicobacter pylori) are a common cause of stomach ulcers, which can sometimes lead to stomach cancer and lymphoma. For a century, physicians refused to believe bacteria caused ulcers because they thought bacteria could not live in the acid environment of the stomach. In 2005 the Nobel Prize in Medicine was awarded to two Australian researchers for their 1982 discovery. These stomach bacteria could only be detected by use of special tissue stains. The CDC now claims that H. pylori causes more than 90% of duodenal ulcers and 80% of gastric ulcers. Approximately two-thirds of the world's population is infected with these microbes.

In the past four years there have been medical reports of newly discovered bacteria in serious lymph node disease; in Hodgkin's lymphoma; in cancer of the mouth; and in prostate cancer, to name only a few.

All of these studies prove bacteria can pop up in diseases where they are least expected. Such a caveat is appropriate for doctors who think they know everything about cancer and who pooh-pooh all aspects of cancer microbe research.

A Century of Cancer Microbe Research

Livingston never claimed that she was the discoverer of the microbe of cancer. In her writings she always gave credit to various scientists, some dating back to the nineteenth century, who attempted to prove that bacteria cause cancer. Some of these remarkable researchers include the long-forgotten cancer microbe studies of Scottish obstetrician James Young, Chicago physician John Nuzum, Montana surgeon James Scott, the infamous psychiatrist and cancer researcher Wilhelm Reich, microscopist Raymond Royal Rife, and others too numerous to mention.

This cancer microbe research has been explored in my books *The Cancer Microbe: The Hidden Killer in Cancer, AIDS, and Other Immune Diseases*, 1990 and in Four Women Against Cancer: Bacteria, Cancer, and *The Origin of Life*, 2005 – the story of Livingston, Alexander-Jackson, Diller and Seibert – four outstanding women scientists who attempted to bring the cancer microbe to the attention of a disinterested medical establishment. I was privileged to have met all of these remarkable women, who greatly influenced my own cancer research.

Why is research exploring bacteria in cancer so strongly opposed? Perhaps it poses a threat to the money interests involved in the established and orthodox treatment for cancer. Various forms of cancer treatment include surgery, radiation and chemotherapy. These therapies might have to be reevaluated if it were proven that cancer was an infectious disease.

Suggestions for Further Internet Study

Further information pertaining to cancer microbe research (both pro and con) can be found by Googling: cancer microbe; bacterial pleomorphism; cell wall-deficient bacteria; "alan cantwell"; "virginia livingston"; "Eleanor Alexander-Jackson"; as well as other names and key words mentioned in this communication.

For a list of scientific publications pertaining to the microbiology of cancer, go to the PubMed website hosted by the National Institute of Health (www.ncbi.nlm.nih.gov) and type in "Cantwell AR", "Livingston VW", "Alexander-Jackson E", "Diller IC", "Seibert FB", etc. in the search box.

This short communication is unlikely to convince many health professionals that bacteria cause cancer. However, after four decades of studying cancer microbes in cancerous tissue, I am personally convinced that Dr. Virginia Livingston will one day be vindicated and recognized as one of the greatest medical geniuses of the twentieth century.

Ralph W Moss, cancer advocate and author of The Cancer Industry, notes her passing was "a major loss to the cancer world." In the *Cancer Chronicles #6*, 1990, he writes, "Virginia Livingston was a great person and a great scientist. Sadly, she never received the recognition she deserved in her lifetime. The true scope of her achievements will only become known in years to come."

This report honors the centennial of her birth which takes place on December 28, 2006.

Bibliography (for Dr. Cantwell's article only)

Alexander-Jackson E. A specific type of microorganism isolated from animal and human cancer: bacteriology of the organism. Growth. 1954 Mar;18(1):37-51.

Cantwell AR. Variably acid-fast cell wall-deficient bacteria as a possible cause of dermatologic disease. In, Domingue GJ (Ed). Cell wall-deficient Bacteria. Reading: Addison-Wesley Publishing Co; 1982.pp. 321-360.

Cantwell A. The Cancer Microbe. Los Angeles: Aries Rising Press; 1990.

Cantwell A. Four Women Against Cancer. Los Angeles: Aries Rising Press; 2005.

Diller IC, Diller WF. Intracellular acid-fast organisms isolated from malignant tissues. Trans Amer Micr Soc. 1965; 84:138-148.

Greenberg DE, Ding L, Zelazny AM, Stock F, Wong A, Anderson VL, Miller G, Kleiner DE, Tenorio AR, Brinster L, Dorward DW, Murray PR, Holland SM. A novel bacterium associated with lymphadenitis in a patient with chronic granulomatous disease. PLoS Pathog. 2006 Apr;2(4):e28.Epub 2006 Apr 14.

Hooper SJ, Crean SJ, Lewis MA, Spratt DA, Wade WG, Wilson MJ. Viable bacteria present within oral squamous cell carcinoma tissue. J Clin Microbiol. 2006 May;44(5):1719-25.

Nuzum JW. The experimental production of metastasizing carcinoma of the breast of the dog and primary epithelioma in man by repeated inoculation of a micrococcus isolated from human breast cancer. Surg Gynecol Obstet. 1925; 11;343-352.

Russell W. An address on a characteristic organism of cancer. Br Med J. 1890; 2:1356-1360.

Russell W. The parasite of cancer. Lancet. 1899;1:1138-1141.

Sauter C, Kurrer MO. Intracellular bacteria in Hodgkin's disease and sclerosing mediastinal B-cell lymphoma: sign of a bacterial etiology? Swiss Med Wkly. 2002 Jun 15;132(23-24):312-5.

Scott MJ. The parasitic origin of carcinoma. Northwest Med. 1925;24:162-166.

Seibert FB, Feldmann FM, Davis RL, Richmond IS. Morphological, biological, and immunological studies on isolates from tumors and leukemic bloods. Ann N Y Acad Sci. 1970 Oct 30;174(2):690-728.

Shannon BA, Garrett KL, Cohen RJ. Links between Propionibacterium acnes and prostate cancer. Future Oncol. 2006 Apr;2(2):225-32.Review.

Wuerthele Caspe-Livingston V, Alexander-Jackson E, Anderson JA, et al. Cultural properties and pathogenicity of certain microorganisms obtained from various proliferative and neoplastic diseases. Amer J Med Sci. 1950; 220;628-646.

Wuerthele-Caspe Livingston V, Livingston AM. Demonstration of Progenitor cryptocides in the blood of patients with collagen and neoplastic diseases. Trans NY Acad Sci. 1972; 174 (2):636-654.

Young J. Description of an organism obtained from carcinomatous growths. Edinburgh Med J. 1921; 27:212-221.

Intracellular Parasites

Modified from Wikipedia, Online version: http://en.wikipedia.org/wiki/ Intracellular_parasite, various references cited.

Intracellular parasites are parasitic microorganisms that are capable of growing and reproducing inside the cells of a host. Facultative types can live and reproduce both inside and outside host cells. Some examples are given below

Bacteria	Fungi	Protozoa
Francisella tularensis	Histoplasma capsulatum	Plasmodium
Listeria monocytogenes	Cryptococcus neoformans	Toxoplasma gondii
Salmonella typhi		
Brucella		
Legionella		
Mycobacterium		
Nocardia		
Rhodococcus equi		
Yersinia		
Neisseria meningitidis		

Obligate intracellular parasites cannot reproduce outside host cells; they must depend on factors within a cell to reproduce. This category includes viruses, but other examples are listed below.

Bacteria	Fungi	Protozoa
Chlamydia	Pneumocystis jirovecii	Apicomplexans, such as Plasmodium species
Rickettsia		
Coxiella		Toxoplasma gondii
Mycobacterium, such as Mycobacterium leprae		Cryptosporidium parvum
		Trypanosomatids, such as Leishmania species
		Trypanosoma cruzi

Bacteria and cancer: cause, coincidence or cure?

by D L Mager (dmager@forsyth.org), *Journal of Translational Medicine* 2006, 4:14 doi:10.1186/1479-5876-4-14. (electronic version online: http://www.translational-medicine.com/content/4/1/14.

Research has found that certain bacteria are associated with human cancers. Their role, however, is still unclear. Convincing evidence links some species to carcinogenesis while others appear promising in the diagnosis, prevention or treatment of cancers. The complex relationship between bacteria and humans is demonstrated by Helicobacter pylori and Salmonella typhi infections. Research has shown that H. pylori can cause gastric cancer or MALT lymphoma in some individuals. In contrast, exposure to H. pylori appears to reduce the risk of esophageal cancer in others. Salmonella typhi infection has been associated with the development of gallbladder cancer; however S. typhi is a promising carrier of therapeutic agents for melanoma, colon and bladder cancers. Thus bacterial species and their roles in particular cancers appear to differ among different individuals. Many species, however, share an important characteristic: highly site-specific colonization. This critical factor may lead to the development of non-invasive diagnostic tests, innovative treatments and cancer vaccines....

It is estimated that over 15% of malignancies worldwide can be attributed to infections or about 1.2 million cases per year. Infections involving viruses, bacteria and schistosomes have been linked to higher risks of malignancy. Although viral infections have been strongly associated with cancers, bacterial associations are significant. For example, convincing evidence has linked Helicobacter pylori with both gastric cancer and mucosa-associated lymphoid tissue (MALT) lymphoma, however other species associated with cancers include: Salmonella typhi and gallbladder cancer, Streptococcus bovis and colon cancer, and Chlamydia pneumoniae with lung cancer. Important mechanisms by which bacterial agents may induce carcinogenesis include chronic infection, immune evasion and immune suppression.

It has been shown that several bacteria can cause chronic infections or produce toxins that disturb the cell cycle resulting in altered cell growth. The resulting damage to DNA is similar to that caused by carcinogenic agents as the genes that are altered control normal cell division and apoptosis....

The immune system is an important line of defense for tumor formation of malignancies that express unique antigens. Certain bacterial infections may evade the immune system or stimulate immune responses that contribute to carcinogenic changes through the stimulatory and mutagenic effects of cytokines released by inflammatory cells....Chronic stimulation of these substances along with environmental factors such as smoking, or a susceptible host appears to contribute significantly to carcinogenesis.

How bacteria could cause cancer: one step at a time

Alistair J. Lax and Warren Thomas, Dept of Oral Microbiology, King's College London, Guy's Hospital, London, UK SE1 9RT, *Trends in Microbiology*, Volume 10, Issue 6, 293-299, 1 June 2002, doi:10.1016/S0966-842X(02)02360-0, Copyright © 2002 Elsevier Science Ltd., All rights reserved.

Abstract

Helicobacter pylori highlighted the potential for bacteria to cause cancer. It is becoming clear that chronic infection with other bacteria, notably Salmonella typhi, can also facilitate tumour development. Infections caused by several bacteria (Bartonella spp., Lawsonia intracellularis and Citrobacter rodentium) can induce cellular proliferation that can be reversed by antibiotic treatment. Other chronic bacterial infections have the effect of blocking apoptosis. However, the underlying cellular mechanisms are far from clear. Conversely, several bacterial toxins interfere with cellular signalling mechanisms in a way that is characteristic of tumour promoters. These include Pasteurella multocida toxin, which uniquely acts as a mitogen, and Escherichia coli cytotoxic necrotizing factor, which activates Rho family signalling. This leads to activation of

COX2, which is involved in several stages of tumour development, including inhibition of apoptosis. Such toxins could provide valuable models for bacterial involvement in cancer, but more significantly they could play a direct role in cancer causation and progression.

Editor: Thanks to Helen Faria, Admin, HaciendaPublishing.com, Former Managing Editor, *Medical Sentinel* for permission to include the following article in this section. The article is available online at http://www.haciendapub.com/medicalsentinel/mycoplasmal-infections-chronic-illnesses-fibromyalgia-and-chronic-fatigue-syndromes-.

Mycoplasmal Infections in Chronic Illnesses: Fibromyalgia and Chronic Fatigue Syndromes, Gulf War Illness, HIV-AIDS and Rheumatoid Arthritis

Author: Garth L. Nicolson, PhD, Marwan Y. Nasralla, PhD, Joerg Haier, MD, PhD, Robert Erwin, MD, Nancy L. Nicolson, PhD, Richard Ngwenya, MD

This article was published in the *Medical Sentinel*, Volume 4, Number 5, September/October 1999, pp. 172-175, 191

Abstract

Invasive bacterial infections are associated with several acute and chronic illnesses, including: aerodigestive diseases such as Asthma, Pneumonia, Inflammatory Bowel Diseases; rheumatoid diseases, such as Rheumatoid Arthritis (RA); immunosuppression diseases such as HIV-AIDS; genitourinary infections and chronic fatigue illnesses such as Chronic Fatigue Syndrome (CFS), Fibromyalgia Syndrome (FMS) and Gulf War Illnesses (GWI). It is now apparent that such infections could be (a) causative, (b) cofactors or (c) opportunistic agents in a variety of chronic illnesses. Using Forensic Polymerase Chain Reaction we have looked for the presence of one class of invasive infection (mycoplasmal infections) inside blood leukocyte samples from patients with CFS (Myalgic Encephalomyelitis), FMS, RA, and GWI. There was a significant difference between symptomatic CFS, FMS, GWI, and RA patients with positive mycoplasmal infections of any species (45-63%) and healthy positive controls (~9%) ($P<0.001$). This difference was even greater when specific species (M. fermentans, M. hominis, M. penetrans, M. pneumoniae) were detected. Except for GWI, most patients had multiple mycoplasmal infections (more than one species of mycoplasma). Patients with different diagnoses but overlapping signs and symptoms often have mycoplasmal infections, and such mycoplasma-positive patients generally respond to multiple cycles of particular antibiotics (doxycycline, minocycline, ciprofloxacin, azithromycin, and clarithromycin). Multiple cycles of these antibiotics plus nutritional support appear to be necessary for successful treatment. In addition, immune enhancement and other supplements appear to help these patients regain their health. Other chronic infections may also be involved to various degrees with or without mycoplasmal infections in causing patient morbidity in various chronic illnesses.

Introduction: Chronic Illnesses

There is growing awareness that many chronic illnesses may have an infectious nature that is either responsible (causative) for the illness, a cofactor for the illness or appears as an opportunistic infection(s) that is responsible for aggravating patient morbidity.(1) There are several reasons for this notion, including the nonrandom or clustered appearance of an illness, often in immediate family members, the course of the illness, and its response to therapies based on infectious agents. Since chronic illnesses are often complex, involving multiple, nonspecific, overlapping signs and symptoms, they are difficult to diagnose and even more difficult to treat. Most chronic illnesses do not have effective therapies, and patients rarely recover from their conditions,(2) causing in some areas of the world catastrophic economic problems.

Some chronic illnesses, such as Rheumatoid Arthritis (RA), are well established in their clinical diagnosis,(3) whereas others, such as Chronic Fatigue Syndrome (CFS, sometimes called Myalgic Encephalomyelitis), Fibromyalgia Syndrome (FMS), and Gulf War Syndrome or Gulf War Illnesses (GWI), have rather nonspecific but similar complex, multi-organ signs and symptoms that overlap or are almost identical.(1) In the case of CFS, FMS and GWI these include: chronic fatigue, headaches, muscle pain and soreness, nausea, gastrointestinal problems, joint pain and soreness, lymph node pain, cognitive problems, depression, breathing problems and other signs and symptoms.(4) The major difference between these illnesses appears to be in the severity of specific signs and symptoms. For example, FMS patients have as their major complaint muscle and overall pain, soreness and weakness, whereas CFS patients most often complain of chronic fatigue and joint pain, stiffness and soreness, but otherwise their complaints usually overlap. Often these patients have increased sensitivities to various environmental irritants and enhanced allergic responses. Although chronic fatigue illnesses have been known for several years, most patients with CFS, FMS, GWI and in some cases RA have had few treatment options. This may have been due to the imprecise nature of their diagnoses, which are based primarily on clinical observations rather than laboratory tests, and a lack of understanding about the underlying causes of these illnesses or the factors responsible for patient morbidity.(1) These illnesses could have different initial causes or triggers but similar cofactors or similar opportunistic infections that cause significant morbidity.

Chronic Illnesses: Overlapping Signs and Symptoms

The multiple signs and symptoms of FMS, CFS and GWI are complex, nonspecific and completely overlapping (Figure 1), suggesting that these illnesses are related and not completely separate syndromes.(1,6) In this figure only differences in the signs and symptoms after the onset of illness are shown, and the data for FMS and CFS have been combined, because previous studies indicated that with the exception of muscle pain and tenderness, there was essentially no difference in patient signs.(4) Illness Survey Forms were analyzed to determine the most common signs and symptoms at the time when blood was drawn from patients. The intensity of patient signs and symptoms prior to and after onset of illness was recorded on a 10-point rank scale (0-10, extreme). The data were arranged by 38 different signs and symptoms and were considered positive if the value after onset of illness was two or more points higher than prior to the onset of illness. The data in Figure 1 indicate that patients diagnosed with CFS or FMS had complex signs and symptoms that were similar to those reported for GWI. In addition, the presence of rheumatoid signs and symptoms in each of these disorders indicates that there are also similarities to RA.(7) Moreover, it is not unusual to find immediate family members who display similar signs and symptoms. For example, there is evidence that GWI has slowly spread to immediate family members,(8) and it is likely that it has also spread to some degree in the workplace.(1) A preliminary survey of approximately 1,200 GWI families indicated that approximately 77% of spouses and a majority of children born after the war had signs and symptoms similar or identical to veterans with GWI.(8)

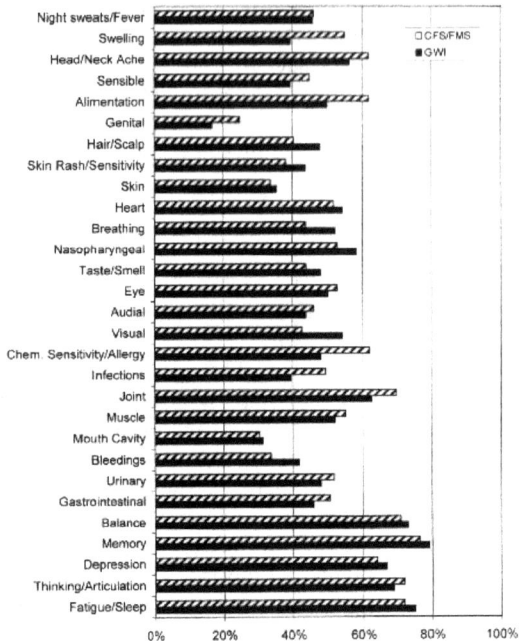

Figure 10: Incidence of increase in severity of signs and symptoms in 203 patients with CFS/FMS compared in GWI after the onset of illness.

Severity was assessed using a Patient Illness Survey Form that included 114 signs and symptoms. The intensity was scored by patients on a 10-point scale (0, none; 10, extreme) prior to and after the onset of illness. Scores were determined in each category (3-9 questions) as the sum of differences between values prior to and after onset of illness divided by the number of questions in the category. Changes in score values of 2 or more points were considered relevant.

In the absence of laboratory tests to the contrary, chronic illnesses are often misdiagnosed as somatoform disorders caused by stress and other nonorganic factors.(9) Patients with CFS, FMS and GWI usually have cognitive problems, such as short term memory loss, difficulty concentrating and other problems, and physicians who find psychological or psychiatric problems in these patients often decide that these conditions are caused by somatoform disorders, not organic problems.(1) Stress is often mentioned as an important factor or the important factor in these disorders. Indeed, GWI patients are often diagnosed with Post Traumatic Stress Disorder (PTSD) in veterans' and military hospitals.(10) The evidence that has been offered as proof that stress or PTSD is the source of GWI sickness is the assumption that veterans must have suffered from stress by virtue of the stressful environment in which they found themselves during the Gulf War,(10) but the veterans themselves do not feel that stress-related diagnoses are an accurate portrayal of their illnesses. Most testimony to date refutes the notion that stress is the major factor in GWI,(11) suggesting that stress, albeit important, is not the cause of GWI.(12) But most physicians would agree that stress can exacerbate chronic illnesses and suppress immune systems, suggesting that stress plays a secondary not primary role in chronic illnesses, such as GWI, CFS, and FMS.(1) However, in the absence of physical or laboratory tests that can identify possible origins of FMS, CFS or GWI, many physicians accept that stress is the cause of these chronic illnesses. It has been only recently that other causes were seriously considered, including chronic infections.(13)

Mycoplasmal Infections in CFS, FMS and GWI

We have been particularly interested in the association of certain chronic infectious agents in CFS, FMS and GWI, because these microorganisms can potentially cause most or essentially all of the signs and symptoms found in these patients.(1,14) One type of infection that elicited our attention was microorganisms of the class Molecutes, small bacterial mycoplasmas, lacking cell walls, that are capable of invading several types of human cells and are associated with a wide variety of human diseases.(14)

We have examined the presence of mycoplasmal blood infections in GWI, CFS, and FMS patients. The clinical diagnosis of these disorders was obtained from referring physicians according to the patients' major signs and symptoms. Since the signs and symptoms of CFS and FMS patients completely overlapped, these patients were therefore considered together (CFS/FMS).(1) Blood was collected, shipped over night at 4°C and processed immediately for PCR after purification of DNA using a Chelex procedure.(1,7) Patients' blood was analyzed for the presence of mycoplasmal infections in blood leukocytes. Positive PCR results were confirmed if the PCR product was 717 base pairs in size using the genus-specific primers (or 850 base pairs for M. fermentans specific primers, etc.) along with a positive control of the same size in the same gel, and if a visible band was obtained after hybridization with the internal probe.(15)

The sensitivity and specificity of the PCR methods were determined by examining serial dilutions of purified DNA of M. fermentans, M. pneumoniae, M. penetrans, M. hominis and M. genetalium. Amounts as low as 10 fg of purified DNA were detectable for all species using the genus primers. The amplification with genus primers produced the expected fragment size in all tested species, which was confirmed by hybridization with an inner probe.(16)

Mycoplasma tests were performed on all patients as described previously (1,7,17) either from Chelex-purified DNA or DNA prepared from whole blood using a commercial kit. The targeted Mycoplasma spp. sequence was amplified from DNA extracted from the peripheral blood of 144/203 CFS or FMS patients (~70%). In 70 healthy subjects positive results for Mycoplasma spp. were obtained in 6 samples (<9%). The difference between patient and control groups was significant (p<0.001).(17) In addition, two of the 70 controls were positive for M. fermentans. The ratio between positive and negative patients was comparable in female and male patients. These results are quite similar to the results recently published by others.(18) Similarly, using Nucleoprotein Gene Tracking to analyze the blood leukocytes from GWI patients we found that 91/200 (45%) were positive for mycoplasmal infections.(19,20) In contrast, in nondeployed, healthy adults the incidence of mycoplasmal infections was 4/62 (~6%).(19,20)

Patients with FMS or CFS often have multiple mycoplasmal infections and probably other chronic infections as well. When we examined CFS/FMS patients for M. fermentans, M. pneumoniae, M. penetrans, M. hominis infections, multiple infections were found in over one-half of 93 patients (Figure 2). CFS/FMS patients had double (over 30%) or triple (over 20%) mycoplasmal infections, but only when one of the species was M. fermentans or M. pneumoniae.(17) Higher score values for increases in the severity of signs and symptoms were also found in patients with multiple infections. CFS/FMS patients infected with different mycoplasma species generally had a longer history of illness, suggesting that patients may have contracted additional infections with time.(17)

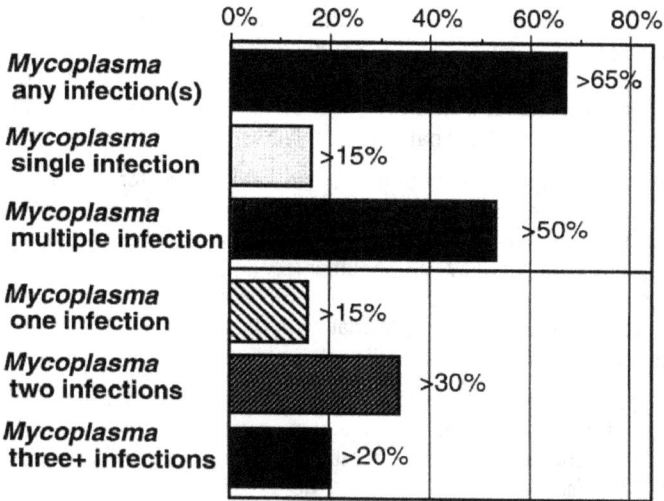

Figure 11: Incidence of multiple mycoplasmal infections in 93 CFS/FMS patients. Patients were examined for M. fermentans, M. pneumoniae, M. penetrans, or M. hominis blood infections by Forensic PCR.

In the course of our studies we found that DNA preparation and blood storage was extremely important in preserving the test samples. Storage of blood frozen or at 0-4°C resulted in reproducible assay results, whereas storage at room temperature resulted in loss of PCR signal over time. Within 1-2 days at room temperature, most of the positive samples reverted to negative results.(1) Also, blood drawn in tubes (blue-top) containing citrate and kept at 0-4°C before the assay yielded better results than other anticoagulants, unless the samples were frozen in EDTA (purple-top) tubes.

Mycoplasmal Infections in Rheumatoid Diseases

The underlying causes of rheumatoid diseases are not known, but RA and other autoimmune diseases could be triggered or exacerbated by infectious agents. It has been known for some time that infectious diseases in some animal species result in remarkable clinical and pathological similarities to RA and other rheumatoid diseases. Aerobic and anaerobic intestinal bacteria, viruses and mycoplasmas have been proposed as important agents in RA.(21) Recently there has been increasing evidence that mycoplasmas may play a role in the initiation or progression of RA.(22) Mycoplasmas have been proposed to interact nonspecifically with B-lymphocytes, resulting in modulation of immunity, autoimmune reactions and promotion of rheumatoid diseases.(23) M. pneumoniae, M. salivarium and U. urealyticum have also been found in the joint tissues of patients with rheumatological diseases, suggesting their pathogenic involvement.(24)

When we examined RA patients' blood leukocytes for the presence of mycoplasmas, we found that approximately one-half were infected with various species of mycoplasmas.(7) The most common species found was M. fermentans, followed by M. pneumoniae and M. hominis and finally M. penetrans. Similar to what we found in CFS/FMS patients, there was a high percentage of multiple mycoplasmal infections in RA patients when one of the species was M. fermentans.(7)

Although the precise role of mycoplasmas in RA and other rheumatoid inflammatory diseases remains unknown, mycoplasmas could be important cofactors in the development of inflammatory responses and for progression of the disease. As an example of the possible role of mycoplasmas in rheumatological diseases, M. arthritidis infections in animals can trigger and exacerbate autoimmune arthritis.(25) This mycoplasma can also suppress T-cells and release substances that act on polymorphonuclear granulocytes, such as oxygen radicals, chemotactic factors, and other substances.(26) Mycoplasmal infections can increase proinflammatory cytokines, such as Interleukin-1, -2, and -6,(27) suggesting that they are involved in the development and possibly progression of rheumatological diseases.

In addition to mycoplasmal infections, other microorganisms have been under investigation as cofactors or causative agents in rheumatological diseases. The discovery of EB virus(28) and cytomegalovirus(29) in the cells of the synovial lining in RA patients suggested their involvement in RA, possibly as a cofactor. There are a number of bacteria and viruses that are candidates in the induction of RA or its progression.(30) In support of bacterial involvement in RA, it has been known for some time that antibiotics like minocycline can alleviate the clinical signs and symptoms of RA.(31) Although this has been proposed to be due to their anti-inflammatory activities, these drugs are likely to be acting to suppress infections of sensitive microorganisms like mycoplasmas.

Mycoplasmal Infections in Immunosuppressive and Autoimmune Diseases

Mycoplasmas have been implicated in the progression of HIV-AIDS. It has been known for some time that some species of mycoplasmas are associated with certain terminal human diseases, such as an acute fatal illness found with certain Mycoplasma fermentans infections in non-AIDS patients.(32) Recently, mycoplasmal infections have attracted attention as a major source of morbidity in AIDS patients. For example, M. fermentans can cause renal and CNS complications in patients with AIDS,(33) and M. penetrans has also been found in the respiratory epithelial cells of AIDS patients.(34) Other species of mycoplasmas have also been found in AIDS patients where they have been associated with disease progression, such as M. prium and M. hominis.(32) Blanchard and Montagnier(35) have proposed that mycoplasmas are cofactors in HIV-AIDS, accelerating progression and accounting, at least in part, for increased susceptibility of AIDS patients to additional infections. In addition to immune suppression, some of this increased susceptibility may be the result of mycoplasma-induced host cell membrane damage from toxic oxygenated products released from intracellular mycoplasmas.(36) Also, mycoplasmas may regulate HIV-LTR-dependent gene expression,(37) suggesting that mycoplasmas may play an important regulatory role in HIV pathogenicity.

There is some preliminary evidence that mycoplasmal infections could be associated with autoimmune diseases. In some mycoplasma-positive GWI cases the signs and symptoms of Multiple Sclerosis (MS), Amyotrophic Lateral Sclerosis (ALS or Lou Gehrig's Disease), Lupus, Graves' Disease and other complex autoimmune diseases have been seen. Such usually rare autoimmune responses are consistent with certain chronic infections, such as mycoplasmal infections, that penetrate into nerve cells, synovial cells and other cell types. These autoimmune signs and symptoms could be caused when intracellular pathogens, such as mycoplasmas, escape from cellular compartments and incorporate into their own structures pieces of host cell membranes that contain important host membrane antigens that can trigger autoimmune responses. Alternatively, mycoplasma surface components ('superantigens') may directly stimulate autoimmune responses,(38) or their molecular mimicry of host antigens may explain, in part, their ability to stimulate autoimmunity.(39)

Mycoplasmal Infections in Other Clinical Conditions

Asthma, airway inflammation, chronic pneumonia and other respiratory diseases are known to be associated with mycoplasmal infections. For example, M. pneumoniae is a common cause of upper respiratory infections,(40) and severe asthma is commonly associated with mycoplasmal infections.(41) Recent evidence has shown that certain mycoplasmas, such as M. fermentans (incognitus strain), are unusually invasive and often found within respiratory epithelial cells.(34)

Heart infections (myocarditis, endocarditis, pericarditis and others) are often due to chronic infections, such as Mycoplasma,(42,43) Chlamydia(44) and possibly other infectious agents.

Other species of mycoplasmas are also associated with various illnesses: M. hominis infections were first found in patients with hypogammaglobulinemia, and M. genitalium was first isolated from the urogenital tracts of patients with nongonococcal urethritis.(45,46) Although mycoplasmas can exist in the oral cavity and gut as normal flora, when they penetrate into the blood and tissues, they may be able to cause or promote a variety of acute or chronic illnesses. These cell-penetrating species, such as M. penetrans, M. fermentans and M. pirum among others, can probably result in complex systemic signs and symptoms. Mycoplasmas are also very effective at evading the immune system, and synergism with other infectious agents can occur.(14) Similar types of chronic infectious agents may occur.(14) Similar types of chronic infections caused by Chlamydia, Brucella, Coxiella or Borrelia may also be present either as single agents or as complex, multiple in

Mycoplasmal Infections: Treatment Suggestions

Once mycoplasmal infections have been identified in the white blood cell fractions of subsets of CFS, FMS, GWI, RA and other patients, they can be successfully treated. Appropriate treatment with antibiotics should result in patient improvement and even recovery.(6,19,20) The recommended treatments for mycoplasmal blood infections require long-term antibiotic therapy, usually multiple 6-week cycles of doxycycline (200-300 mg/day),(47) ciprofloxacin (1,500 mg/day), azithromycin (500 mg/day) or clarithromycin (750-1,000 mg/day).(48) Multiple cycles are required, because few patients recover after only a few cycles, possibly because of the intracellular locations of mycoplasmas like M. fermentans and M. penetrans, the slow-growing nature of these microorganisms and their relative drug sensitivities. For example, of 87 GWI patients that tested positive for mycoplasmal infections, all patients relapsed after the first 6-week cycle of antibiotic therapy, but after up to 6 cycles of therapy 69/87 patients recovered and returned to active duty.(19,20) The clinical responses that were seen were not due to placebo effects, because administration of some antibiotics, such as penicillins, resulted in patients becoming more not less symptomatic, and they were not due to immunosuppressive effects that can occur with some of the recommended antibiotics. Interestingly, CFS, FMS and GWI patients that slowly recover after several cycles of antibiotics are generally less environmentally sensitive, suggesting that their immune systems may be returning to pre-illness states. If such patients had illnesses that were caused by psychological or psychiatric problems or solely by chemical exposures, they should not respond to the recommended antibiotics and slowly recover. In addition, if such treatments were just reducing autoimmune responses, then patients should relapse after the treatments are discontinued.(1)

Patients with CFS, FMS, RA or GWI usually have nutritional and vitamin deficiencies that must be corrected.(48) These patients are often depleted in vitamins B, C, and E and certain minerals. Unfortunately, patients with these chronic illnesses often have poor absorption. Therefore, high doses of some vitamins must be used, and others, such as vitamin B complex, must be given sublingual. Antibiotics that deplete normal gut bacteria can result in over-growth of less desirable flora, so Lactobacillus acidophillus supplementation is recommended. In addition, a number of natural remedies that boost the immune system are available and are potentially useful, especially during antibiotic therapy or after therapy has been completed.(48) One of us (R.N.) has been involved in the development of ancient African and Chinese natural immune enhancers and cleansers help to restore natural immunity and absorption. Although these products are known to help AIDS patients, their clinical effectiveness in GWI/CFS/FMS/RA patients has not been carefully evaluated. They appear to be useful during therapy to boost the immune system or after antibiotic therapy in a maintenance program to prevent relapses.(48)

Why aren't physicians routinely treating mycoplasmal and other chronic infections? In many cases they are treating these infections, but it has been only recently that such infections have been found in so many unexplained chronic illnesses. These infections cannot be successfully treated with the usual short courses of antibiotics due to their intracellular locations, slow proliferation rates and inherent insensitivity to most antibiotics. In addition, a fully functional immune system may be essential to overcoming these infections, and this is why vitamin and nutritional supplements are so important.

Conclusions

We have proposed that chronic infections are an appropriate explanation for the morbidity seen in a rather large subset of CFS, FMS, GWI and RA patients, and in a variety of other illnesses. Not every patient will have this as a diagnostic explanation or have the same types of chronic infections, and additional research is necessary to clarify the role of such infections in chronic diseases.(1,7) Some patients may have chemical or radiological exposures or other environmental problems as an underlying reason for their chronic signs and symptoms. In these patients, chronic infections may be opportunistic. In others, somatoform disorders or illnesses caused by psychological or psychiatric problems may indeed be important. However, in these patients antibiotics, supplements and immune enhancers should have no lasting effect whatsoever, and they should not recover on such therapies. **The identification of specific infectious agents in the blood of chronically ill patients may allow many patients with CFS, FMS, GWI or RA and other chronic diseases to obtain more specific diagnoses and effective treatments for their illnesses. Finally, patients with cardiopathies, AIDS, respiratory illnesses, and urogenital infections are often infected with Mycoplasma, Chlamydia, Brucella or other chronic, invasive bacterial and parasitic infections, and these patients could benefit from appropriate antibiotic and neutraceutical therapies that alleviate morbidity.**

References

1. Nicolson GL, Nasralla M, Haier J, Nicolson NL. Biomed. Therapy 1998;16:266-271.

2. Hoffman C, Rice D, Sung H-Y. (1996) JAMA 1996;276:1473-1479.

3. Hochberg MC, et al. Arthritis Rheumatol. 1992;35:498-502.

4. Nicolson GL, Nicolson NL. J. Occup. Environ. Med. 1996;38:14-16.

5. Murray-Leisure K. et al. Intern. J. Med. 1998;1:47-72.

6. Nicolson GL. Intern. J. Med. 1998;1:42-46.

7. Haier J, Nasralla M, Nicolson GL. Rheumatol 1999;38:504-509.

8. Senate Committee on Banking, Housing and Urban Affairs, U. S. Congress (1994) U.S. chemical and biological warfare-related dual use exports to Iraq and their possible impact on the health consequences of the Persian Gulf War, 103rd Congress, 2nd Session, Report: May 25, 1994.

9. N.I.H. Technology Assessment Workshop Panel. The Persian Gulf experience and health. JAMA 1994;272:391-396.

10. Nicolson GL, Nicolson NL. Med. Confl. Surviv. 1997;13:140-146.

11. House Committee on Government Reform and Oversight, U. S. Congress (1997) Gulf War veterans': DOD continue to resist strong evidence linking

toxic causes to chronic health effects, 105th Congress, 1st Session, Report: 105-388.

12. U. S. General Accounting Office (1997) Gulf War Illnesses: improved monitoring of clinical progress and reexamination of research emphasis are needed. Report: GAO/SNIAD-97-163.

13. Nicolson GL, Nicolson NL. Townsend Lett. Doctors 1996;156:42-48.

14. Baseman JB, Tully JG. Emerg. Infect. Dis. 1997;3:21-32.

15. Van Kuppeveld FJM, et al. Appl. Environ. Microbiol. 1992;58:2606-2615.

16. Erlich HA, Gelfand D, Sninsky JJ. Science 1991;252:1643-1651.

17. Nasralla M, Haier J, Nicolson GL. Clin. Microbiol. Infect. Dis. 1999; in press.

18. Vojdani A, Choppa PC, Tagle C, Andrin R, Samimi B, Lapp CW. FEMS Immunol. Med. Microbiol. 1998;22:355-365.

19. Nicolson GL, Nicolson NL. Intern. J. Occup. Med. Immunol. Tox. 1996;5:69-78.

20. Nicolson GL, Nicolson NL, Nasralla M. Intern. J. Med. 1998;1:80-92.

21. Midvedt T. Scan. J. Rheumatol. Suppl. 1987;64:49-54.

22. Schaeverbeke T, et al. Rev. Rheumatol. 1997;64:120-128.

23. Simecka JW, Ross SE, Cassell GH, Davis JK. Clin. Infect. Dis. 1993;17 (Supp. 1):S176-S182.

24. Furr PM, Taylor-Robinson D, Webster ADB. Ann. Rheumatol. Dis. 1994;53:183-184.

25. Cole BC, Griffith MM. Arthritis Rheumatol. 1993;36:994-1002.

26. Kirchhoff H, et al. Rheumatol. Int. 1989;9:193-196.

27. Mühlradt PF, Quentmeier H, Schmitt E. Infect. Immunol. 1991;58:1273-1280.

28. Fox RI, Luppi M, Pisa P, Kang HI. J. Rheumatol. 1992;32:18-24.

29. Takei M, et al. Int. Immunol. 1997;9:739-743.

30. Krause A, Kamradt T, Burnmester GR. Curr. Opin. Rheumatol. 1996;8:203-209.

31. Tilley BC, et al. Ann. Intern. Med. 1995;122:81-89.

32. Savio ML, et al. New Microbiol. 1996;19:203-209.

Additional Reading

33. Bauer FA, Wear D J, Angritt P, Lo S-C. Hum. Pathol. 1991;22:63-69.

34. Stadtlander CT, Watson HL, Simecka JW, Cassell GH. Clin. Infect. Dis. 1993;17 (Suppl. 1):S289-S301.

35. Blanchard A, Montagnier L. Ann. Rev. Microbiol. 1994;48:687-712.

36. Pollack J D, Jones MA, Williams MV. Clin. Infect. Dis. 1993;17 (Suppl. 1):S267-S271.

37. Nir-Paz R, Israel S, Honigman A, Kahane I. FEMS Microbiol. Lett. 1995;128:63-68.

38. Kaneoka H, Naito S. Jap. J. Clin. Med. 1997;6:1363-1369.

39. Baseman JB, Reddy SP, Dallo SP. Am. J. Respir. Crit. Care Med. 1996;154:S137-S144.

40. Balassanian N, Robbins FC. N. Engl. J. Med. 1967;277:719.

41. Gill JC, Cedillo RL, Mayagoitia BG, Paz MD. Ann. Allergy 1993;70:23-25.

42. Prattichizzo FA, Simonetti I, Galetta F. Minerva Cardioangiol. 1997;45:447-450.

43. Hofner G, et al. Zeit. Kardiol. 1997;86:423-426.

44. Bowman J, et al. J. Infect. Dis. 1998;178:274-277.

45. Tully JG, Taylor-Robinson D, Cole RM, Rose DL. Lancet 1981;1:1288-1291.

46. Risi GF Jr, Martin DH, Silberman JA, Cohen JC. Mol. Cell. Probes 1987;1:327-335.

47. Nicolson GL, Nicolson NL. JAMA 1995;273:618-619.

48. Nicolson GL. Intern. J. Med. 1998;1:115-117 and 123-128.

Prof. Garth L. Nicolson, Drs. Marwan Nasralla, Joerg Haier, Robert Erwin and Nancy L. Nicolson are affiliated with The Institute for Molecular Medicine, 15162 Triton Lane, Huntington Beach, CA 92649-1401, (714) 903-2900, Fax (714) 379-2082, website: www.immed.org, email: gnicimm@ix.netcom.com; Dr. Richard Ngwenya is affiliated with the James Mobb Immune Enhancement Clinics, 132 Josiah Chinamano Ave., Harare, Zimbabwe, Fax: +263-4-739-832.

Dr. Nicolson et al's article is hereby published as one view of the possible cause(s) of the Gulf War Syndrome and other chronic illnesses and because a federal grant has been earmarked to evaluate his thesis, but its publication should not be construed as an endorsement of that thesis by the Medical Sentinel or the AAPS---Editor.

Additional Reading

Appendix B: Food Supplements

This appendix lists as current information as possible about vendors that provide food supplements described in the text.

Biotics Research Corporation
http://www.bioticsresearch.com/landing/index.php?show=1
6801 Biotics Research Dr
Rosenberg, TX 77471
800-231-5777
281-344-0909 Local
281-344-0725 Fax
http://www.bioticsresearch.com/sfcontactus
http://www.bioticsresearch.com/productlist

Enzyme Process
http://www.enzymeprocess.co/
index.php?option=com_content&view=article&id=100&Itemid=498
470 N. 56th Street
Chandler, Arizona 85226
Toll Free: 800-521-8669
E-mail: info@enzymeprocess.co
http://www.enzymeprocess.co/
index.php?option=com_virtuemart&view=category&virtuemart_catego
ry_id=23&categorylayout=default&virtuemart_manufacturer_id=2&sh
owcategory=1&showproducts=1&productsublayout=0&Itemid=561

Food Supplements

Lily of the Desert http://www.lilyofthedesert.com/ 1887 Geesling Rd. Denton, TX 76208 940-566-9914 (800) 229-5459 Fax: 940-566-9925 http://www.lilyofthedesert.com/contact-us/ http://www.lilyofthedesert.com/our-products/
Life-Mate (Formerly Research Formula #2) http://lifematenutrition.com/ 351 W 6160 S Murray, UT 84107 888-600-1703 http://lifematenutrition.com/contact-us/ http://lifematenutrition.com/why-choose-life-mate/ingredients/
Miller Pharmacals http://www.millerpharmacal.com/index.php Miller Pharmacal Group 350 Randy Road, Suite 2 Carol Stream, IL 60188-1831 (800) 323-2935 Monday through Friday between 7:30 AM - 4:00 PM Central Time http://www.millerpharmacal.com/contact.html http://www.millerpharmacal.com/products.html
Standard Process Inc. http://www.standardprocess.com/ 1200 W. Royal Lee Drive Palmyra, WI 53156 800-848-5061 (toll free) 262-495-2122 (local) Customer Service (Orders) Phone: 800-558-8740 Fax: 800-438-3799 Email: info@standardprocess.com Email: SPOrders@standardprocess.com http://www.standardprocess.com/Standard-Process/Key-Ingredient-Cross-Reference

---

Vitaminerals
http://www.vmmedical.com/
Email: info@VMMedical.com
Email: order@VMMedical.com
http://www.vmmedical.com/vitaminerals_patient_price_list.htm

Food Supplements

Index

Figures

Tables